INGUINAL HERNIA

Edited by **Silvestro Canonico**

Inguinal Hernia
http://dx.doi.org/10.5772/57011
Edited by Silvestro Canonico

Contributors

Andrzej Komorowski, Jose Ramon Martin-Hidalgo Rodil, David Dominguez Usero, Jorge Moran Rodriguez, Selim Sozen, Suleyman Cetinkunar, Hasan Erdem, Seyfi Emir, Caglar Bilgin, Ilhan Bali, Masao Endo, Evangelos Misiakos, Baki Ekçi, Yuri Kozlov, Antonio Marte

Published by InTech

Janeza Trdine 9, 51000 Rijeka, Croatia

Publishing Process Manager Iva Lipovic

Technical Editor InTech DTP team

Cover InTech Design team

First published June, 2014

Printed in Croatia

Additional hard copies can be obtained from orders@intechopen.com

Inguinal Hernia, Edited by Silvestro Canonico

p. cm.

ISBN 978-953-51-1577-9

For EU product safety concerns:
IN TECH d.o.o., Prolaz Marije Krucifikse Kozulić 3, 51000 Rijeka, Croatia,
info@intechopen.com or visit our website at intechopen.com.

Meet the editor

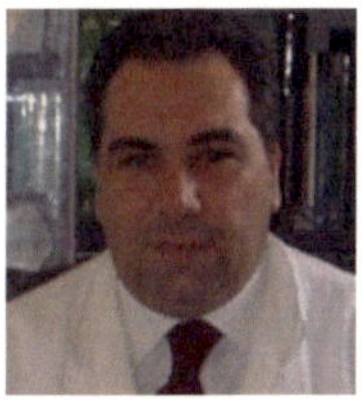

Professor Silvestro Canonico was born in Civitavecchia (Rome, Italy) on the 21st of November 1950 and graduated in Medicine and Surgery magna cum laude at the University of Naples on the 19th of July 1974. He earned the Specialization in Vascular Surgery (08-Jul-1977) and in General Surgery (17-Jun-1982). In 1983 he earned the title of Consultant Surgeon. In 2003 he served as full professor of General Surgery at the Second University of Naples, Italy. He is also serving as : Chief of the Division of General and Geriatric Surgery, University Hospital of the Second University of Naples, Italy; Member of the Academic Senate of the Second University of Naples

Contents

Preface

Hernia was present in human history since its beginning. Groin hernia is already described in the 15th-century Egyptian Papirus of Ebers as swelling that comes out during coughing. In ancient times, Galen contributed much to knowledge of hernia, and his concepts lasted almost unaltered until the Middle Ages and Renaissance. Along with anatomical studies and discoveries, the study of hernia pathophysiology flourished between 18th and 19th century. However, the results of treatment still were largely unsatisfactory.

It became clearer that dealing with the surgical treatment of hernia required an extensive knowledge and technical ability. Astley Cooper stated that no disease of surgical interest requires so broad skills and knowledge as hernia and its variants. Anaesthesia and antisepsis played a pivotal role in the development of groin hernia surgery between 19th and 20th century. In this era the concept of hernia repair under tension was introduced, and mainly relied on antiseptic/aseptic procedures, high ligation of the hernia sac, and narrowing of the internal inguinal ring. These principles did not succeed in obtaining good results, with a 100% recurrence rate within 5 years and postoperative mortality reaching 7%.

Bassini introduced a new *rule* in hernia surgery i.e. the reconstruction of the posterior wall of the inguinal canal, which increased the success rates of surgery. Shouldice later described imbrication of the transverse fascia and strengthening of the posterior wall of the inguinal canal by four layers of fasciae and oblique muscles aponeuroses. By adopting these modifications, recurrence rate fall to 3%.

The principle of *tension free* repair was another landmark of groin hernia surgery. A reduced tension of the sutured layers was achieved by incisions of the rectal abdominal sheath or using foreign materials, which were used widespread after the discovery of synthetic polymers in 1930s. Lichtenstein was the first surgeon to describe a tension free technique by strengthening the posterior wall of inguinal canal with prosthetic material: he published data on 1000 operations with Marlex mesh without recurrences at 5-year follow-up.

Other treatment modalities and techniques have later been described. In 1975 Stoppa proposed placing a mesh in the preperitoneal space without stitches, reporting acceptable recurrences (<2%). In 1968 Lichtenstein used a cigarette-shaped Marlex mesh plug for inguinal and femoral hernias. Prolene was later introduced allowing repair of tissue defect in three spaces: preperitoneal, above the transverse fascia, and inside the inguinal canal.

Besides conventional treatment of groin hernia, the present book is designed to focus on specific topics and problems as well as particular situations which a general surgeon dealing with groin hernia is very likely to face during his practice.

Laparoscopic surgery has gained wide popularity in the 1990s. The laparoscopic treatment of groin hernias began in 1979 when Fletcher performed the first lap repair. Laparoscopic surgery offers several advantages i.e. reducing postoperative pain and the need of wide incisions. It can be very useful in recurrent hernias. Several modifications and advancements have been made since the first lap repair. Schultz introduced the placement of a plug in the inguinal canal with polypropylene mesh in 1990. Then, other techniques were introduced (TEP, TAPP). The increased expertise with the procedure made it suitable also in children presenting with groin hernia, in whom laparoscopy can be very useful. In fact, conventional inguinal hernia open repair in small infants may be technically demanding and is associated with increased risk of incarceration, recurrence and testicular atrophy.

The recent technological advancements allowed extending the indications to minimally invasive repair. The improved instrumentation and the development of biological mesh lead to increase of the surgeon's confidence with the procedure, making it suitable also in incarcerated hernia, allowing a better preservation of the body anatomy. Very recently a technique of laparoscopic transabdominal preperitoneal hernioplasty with mesh fixation by means of human fibrin glue has been introduced (TISTA technique), and provided promising results in terms of reduced postoperative neuralgia and earlier resumption of social and physical activities.

However, laparoscopy brings about some disadvantages, such as the costs of the procedure and the risk due to general anaesthesia. These are discussed, and the advancements in anaesthetic techniques and technological evolution of surgical instrumentation may play a role in reducing their effects.

Special situations are also described in this book. The history of groin hernia repair evolved from life-saving procedures (such as for incarcerated hernias) to elective operations performed as day-surgery procedure. However, acute presentations are still being observed. Strangulated groin hernias could be very difficult to treat, but evidence suggests that both open and laparoscopic approach may be feasible in these situations, provided adequate experience and knowledge have been acquired. Also, the book reports on slipping groin hernias, and presentation and treatment are described.

Lastly, the so-called "sports hernia" or "sportsman's hernia" are described, which present with painful groin in sports involving kicking and twisting movements while running, and can be found also in normally physically active people, usually occurring without a palpable hernia. To avoid confusion, this condition has been recently named "pubic inguinal pain syndrome", and requires different surgical treatments, including the release of the nerves of the inguinal region, the correction of strength imbalance in the muscle structures, and the correction of potential weakness of the posterior inguinal wall.

In conclusion, the aim of this book is to provide the readers with informative and practical indications to understand, diagnose, and manage patients presenting with groin hernia. It could hopefully stimulate further innovative studies and techniques suitable for the treatment of such a common, but often underestimated, condition.

Prof. Silvestro Canonico
Head, Department of Medical, Surgical and Ageing Sciences
Second University of Naples
Naples, Italy

Section 1

Historical Aspects

Chapter 1

History of the Inguinal Hernia Repair

Andrzej L. Komorowski

Additional information is available at the end of the chapter

http://dx.doi.org/10.5772/58533

1. Introduction

1.1. Early attempts at the treatment of inguinal hernia

The inguinal hernia is one of the diseases that haunted the humanity from its very beginning to the modern times. The currently used term „hernia" comes directly from ancient Greece: (kele/hernios in Greek means bud or offshoot). Although the natural course of the disease is relatively slow it eventually reaches the size that severely impairs the patient ability to perform daily activities (Figure 1). That is why already in antique times the surgeons and physicians alike were trying to find the solution for this highly disturbing condition. The mainstay of treatment remained the use of different types of inguinal belts that were supposed to maintain the hernia sac inside the body cavity. To successfully apply the herniary belt the hernia was first manually reduced (Figure 2) and then, the herniary belt, often custom made for a particular patient, was applied. The use of hernia belts was widespread and even today it can be found in some regions of the world.

The wide popularity of the belts was maintained because the surgical option for the cure of inguinal hernia was extremely dangerous and unfortunately not very convincing. One of the first attempts to solve inguinal hernia by the means of surgical knife came from the famous XVIth century Italian anatomist, Gabriele Fallopio. Fallopio proposed wide excision of the sac with surrounding skin and all its contents, securing the neck with an impressive suture (so called the golden stiich). The technique did not become very popular among patients because it resulted in castration and sometimes in the permanent stoma from the cut intestinal loop. The risk of death from bleeding and peritonitis was also important limiting factor of this technique [1]. This is why many barber-surgeons of that time suggested that the operation should be considered „only for marked hernias, which could not be held even with the strongest and surdiest bands at their right place" [2].

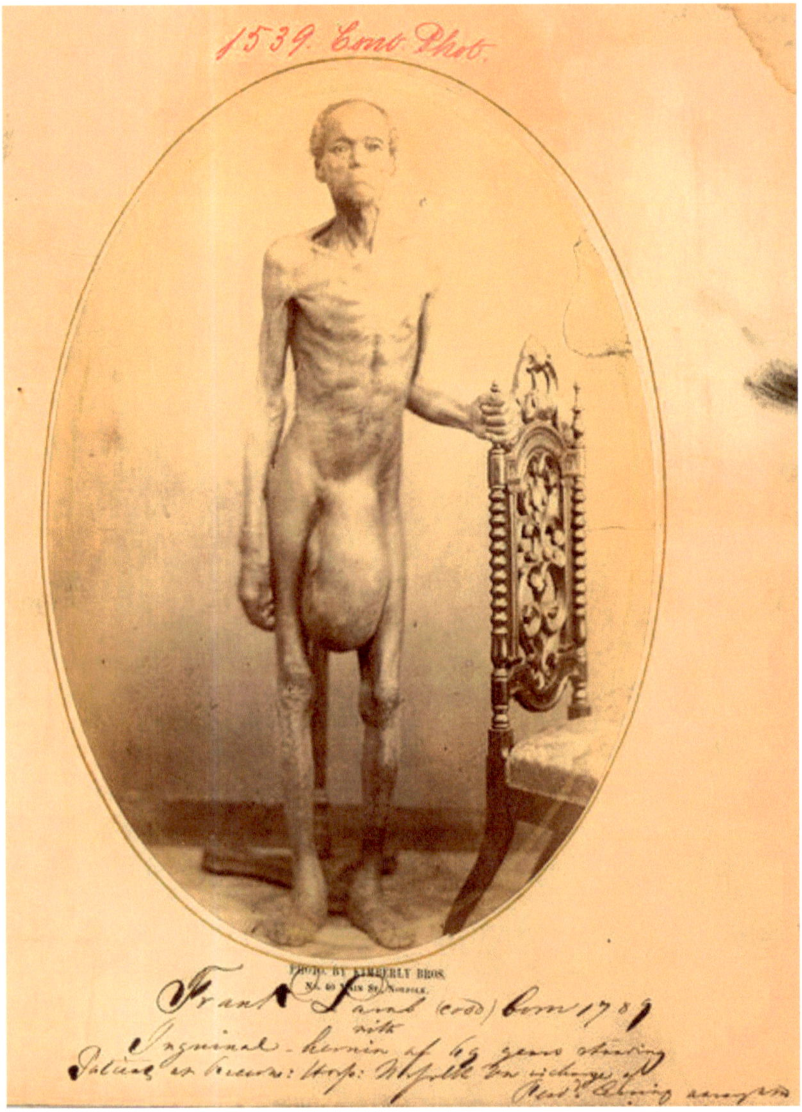

Figure 1. A man with a 69 years history of inguinal hernia. The patient, Frank Lamb, was a slave in North Carolina and since he was 9 years old suffered from left inguinal hernia. Nevertheless he was forced to hard, daily labor. As a result an important inguino-scrotal herniary sac developed. From: Otis Historical Archives of "National Museum of Health and Medicine".

Another worth noticing attempt at giving surgical solution to the inguinal hernia was done by Claudius Amyand from London who in 1735 operated on an 11-year-old boy. The patient suffered from a right inguinal hernia complicated by a faecal fistula. The operation performed by Claudius Amyand is important for two reasons. Firstly, it is the earliest description of a hernia containing a vermiform appendix (known today as Amyand's hernia). And secondly, it is the earliest documented appendicectomy in the history of surgery. On the other hand it

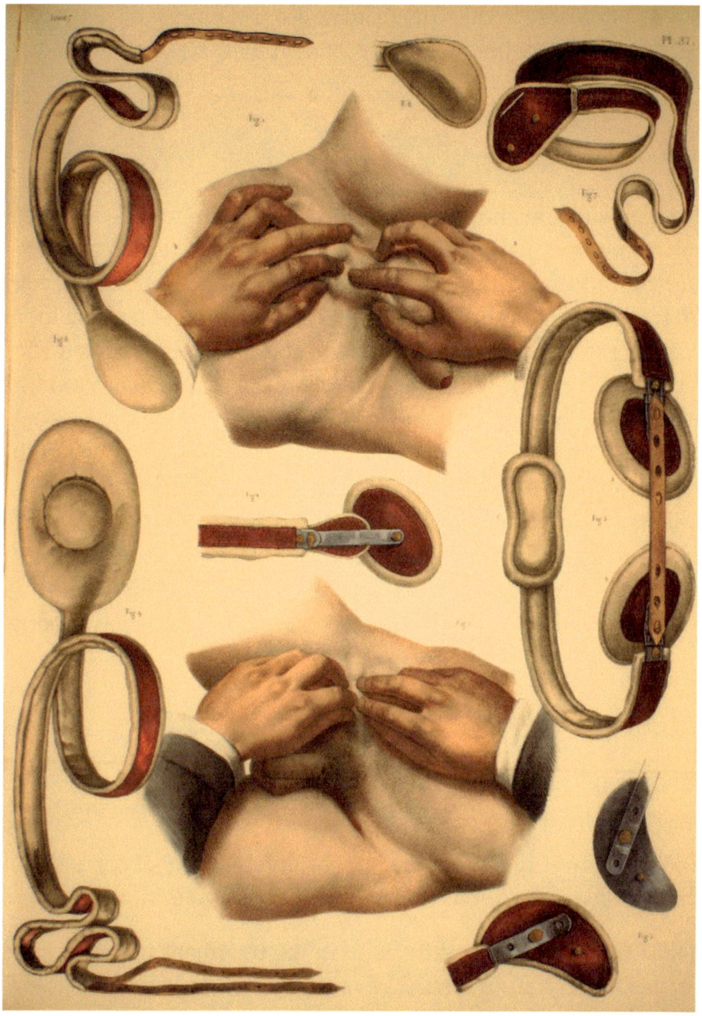

Figure 2. Manual reduction of the inguinal hernia and the use of herniary belts. Image courtesy: BIU Santé (Paris) http://www.biusante.parisdescartes.fr/histmed/image?med02083x07ax0493

shows us that the decision to operate on a hernia patient was made when surgeon was facing a complex problem that required a daredevil solution [3].

The anatomical knowledge of human body was still evolving in XVIIth century. Some advances of the treatment of inguinal hernias, especially incarcerated hernias that posed direct danger of death to the patient if not reduced or operated on has been made in this era. The Spanish anatomist and surgeon Antonio Gimbernat y Arbos after studying anatomy of inguinal canal witnessed an anatomical presentation in London in 1777, performed by famous John Hunter. Gimbernat noticed that Hunter experienced problems in reducing a femoral hernia so he stopped the presentation and told Hunter to cut ligamentum lacunare and this way open femoral canal. After a moment of reflexion Hunter replied: „You're right Sir. I will operate on femoral hernia only in this way from now on." Once again, we have to bear in mind that hernia operations in this era were rare and limited to very desperate, live-or-death situations [4].

1.2. New trends in XIXth century

The fast evolution of medicine and surgery in the XIXth century gave way to some new ideas in the treatment of inguinal hernia. The introduction of antisepsis, asepsis and anesthesia allowed for safer procedures. The advances in anatomical knowledge of hernia lead to the introduction of two important rules for hernia surgery: high ligation of hernia sac and narrowing of the internal inguinal ring. Among techniques that received some fame among XIXth century surgeons we should mention the techniques of William Wood, Vinzenz Czerny and James Heaton. Heaton was performing injection of the mixture of white oak and morphine into the hernia sac to obtain its fibrosis [5]. Czerny was performing the high ligation of the hernia sac and complete closure of the internal inguinal ring with sutures [6]. In the Wood's method the surgeon was supposed to double ligate herniary sac to perform a natural „plug" and use it to close internal inguinal ring [7]. Unfortunately although these techniques looked appealing at first, in the long term virtually all patients experienced hernia recurrence [5]. Let us also remind the reader that the mortality after these operations was reported to be as high as 7% [8].

2. The revolution of Edoardo Bassini

„In order to achieve a radical cure of hernia it is absolutely essential to restore those conditions in the area of the hernial orifice, which exist under normal conditions"-Edoardo Bassini.

It wasn't until 1887 that the real breakthrough in the treatment of inguinal hernia came. All started with a young student from Pavia University, Edoardo Bassini entering in the ranks of Giuseppe Garibaldi's army. During the battle against papal guards near Villa Glori in Rome, Bassini received a bayonet wound in his right groin. After remaining unconscious in the battlefield for several hours he finally recovered only to find out that the bayonet has penetrated the intestinal wall and the coecal fistula has formed within the wound. He turned for help to his university professor Luigi Porta and remained a patient in Pavia for almost 6 months. The coecostomy finally closed but during that time Bassini studied extensively the anatomy and physiology of the inguinal region. Afterwards he started to perform inguinal hernia operation with the techniques of Wood and Heaton but all operated hernias recurred. At this point Bassini realized that the problem was more within the diseased anatomy and physiology of the inguinal canal than in the technique itself. Therefore he come up with the idea that only complete reconstruction of the anatomy of the inguinal canal can lead to a full recovery from inguinal hernia [5]. The meticulous anatomical knowledge led to a surgical technique that Bassini applied with important success to his patients in Padua, where he started to practice after graduation. Bassini has presented his first results in Padua in Italian during surgical congress in Genoa [9] and after a few years in German to gain a wider audience [10].

Within few years his original method (Figure 3) become a classic. His achievement is even more impressive if we realize that all subsequent methods of inguinal hernia surgery until introduction of artificial materials were in fact variants of Bassini concept. The popularization of the Bassini technique was so successful because it was a breakthrough concept but also because Bassini's pupils (among them Atillo Catterina) have done a lot to promote his achievements [11].

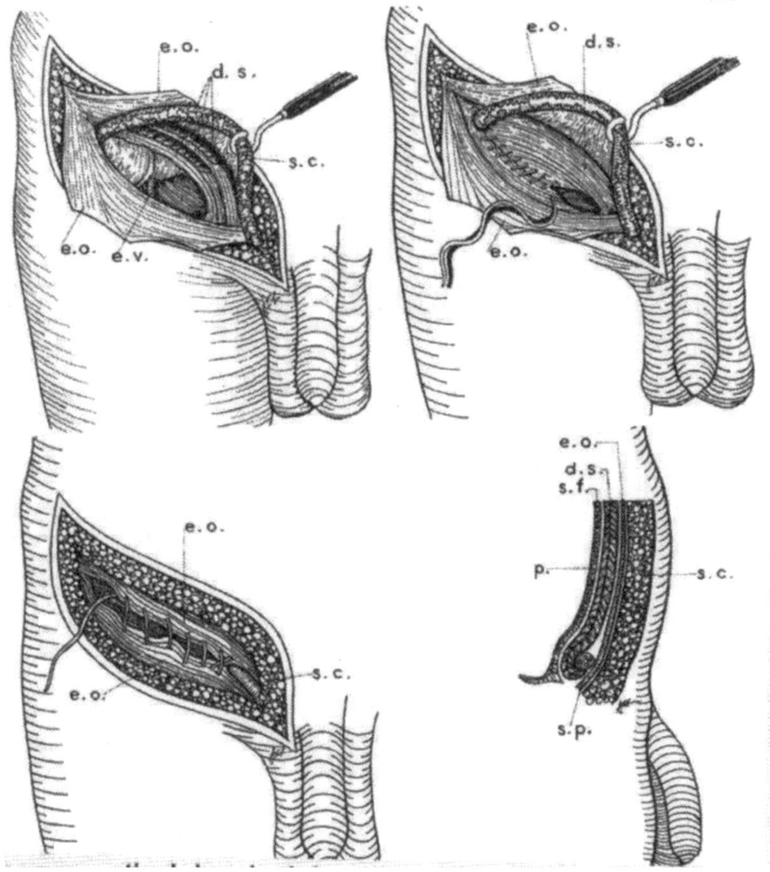

Figure 3. The schematic drawing of the Bassini technique from the German version of his original publication: Ueber de bechandlung des Leistenbruches. Archiv fur Klinische Chirurgie 1890;40:429 [10]

2.1. William Steward Halsted's method and other variants of Bassini's approach.

The main difference of Halsted proposition from Bassini method was the localization of the spermatic cord. After reconstructing the inguinal canal Halsted was leaving spermatic cord in the subcutaneous position. It allowed for closure of the posterior wall of the inguinal canal with a very strong, transfixing sutures. Unfortunately among the first five patients operated by Halsted himself, one developed urinary fistula due to too deep transfixing sutures that pierced through urinary bladder wall. The fistula eventually closed but it showed clearly the risk of too deep sutures placed in the transverse fascia and in the preperitoneum [12].

The subcutaneous position of the spermatic cord exactly as in the Halsted's method was applied also in several other modifications proposed by several surgeons in the years to come. Among them we would like to cite a method described by Paolo Postempski from Rome (Figure 4) [13].

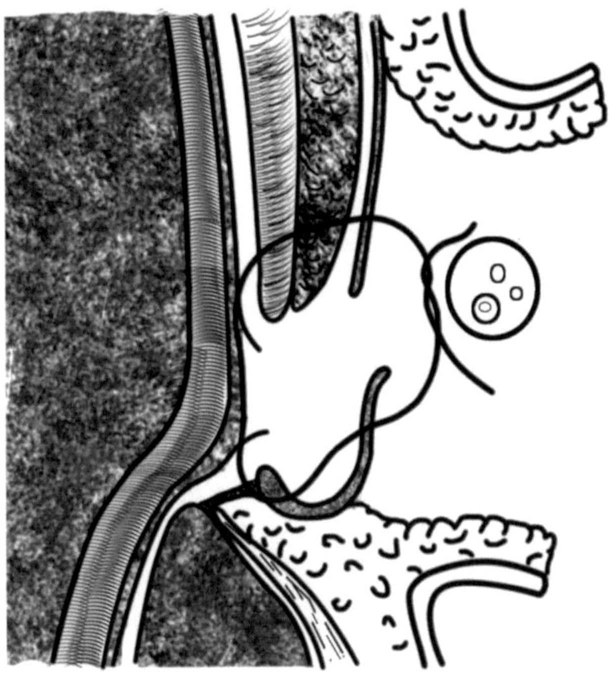

Figure 4. Schematic representation of the Postempski repair. Note subcutaneous position of the spermatic cord as in the Halsted's method. Drawing by dr Jerzy W.Mituś based on Gangeri G. Risorse in chirurgia generale. Kofler Editore, Bassano del Grappa 2006 [12].

Among many variants of Bassini method it would be also interested to mention „The Polish technique" developed by Zdzisław Sławiński in Warsaw and popularized during the World War I. It has gained important fame especially after Sławiński operated with success on cardinal Achille Ratii who later become pope Pio XI. The peculiarity of this technique consisted on dissecting only the neck of the hernia sac, ligating and cutting it and leaving the cut sac „in situ" [14].

At the advent of World War II Chester McVay from Ann Arbor popularized his concept of inguinal hernia repair using Cooper's ligament instead of inguinal ligament as a lower edge of sutures aimed at reconstructing posterior wall of the inguinal canal. In McVay's opinion the use of inguinal ligament by all his predecessors was a „fundamental error" that has led to high hernia recurrence rate [15].

Probably the last big step in the evolution of the „tension" repairs of inguinal hernias was the method described and mastered over the years by Edward Earl Shouldice from Toronto. His idea started in the fifties and was slowly evolving to reach a very mature technique. Shouldice advocated meticulous dissection, complete incision of the transverse fascia, sutures with monofilament rather than silk, oversewing of the posterior wall of inguinal canal by four layers of fascia and aponeuroses of oblique muscles and finally rapid ambulation of the patient (patient were walking home after 2-3 days when at that time it was customary for other surgeons to retain their hernia patients up to 3 weeks in bed). Interestingly there exist no single description of the technique published by Shouldice. Apparently, Shouldice thought that all those willing to learn his technique should come to Toronto and see him performing the famous „Canadian repair". Indeed, the 3% hernia recurrence rate in Shouldice Hernia Hospital was impressive at the time when majority of hospitals experienced even 20% of hernia recurrence. The Shouldice repair can be seen as a final, close to perfect state of Bassini method. As Robert Bendavid stated:"The Shouldice repair, which on occasion is referred to as the Canadian operation, is a derivation of the Bassini repair and incorporates succinct changes, which must be appreciated. It will become evident why Earle Shouldice can be considered the heir to Bassini and to have enhanced that envious stature" [16].

At the advent of wide availability of prosthetic materials the tension repairs have seen a major decline in their use. However, several surgeons see the classic techniques as an interesting and viable option for a selected group of hernia patient. The most popular techniques used until recently (and in some cases even today) include the Bassini, Postempski and Shouldice operations [17]. The major developments in the history of tension repairs of inguinal hernia are shown in the Table 1.

Author	Year	Technique
Edoardo Bassini	1887	reconstructing the anatomy of the inguinal canal
William Steward Halsted	1889	subcutaneous position of the spermatic cord
Paolo Postempski	1890	subcutaneous position of the spermatic cord and closure of external inguinal ring
Zdzisław Sławiński	1916	herniary sac left „in situ", the neck of the sac used to close internal ring
Chester McVay	1942	Cooper's ligament instead of inguinal (Poupart's) ligament for the reconstruction
Edward Earl Shouldice	1953	incision and reconstruction of the transverse fascia

Table 1. Major developments in hernia repair without use of artificial materials (tension techniques)

3. The tension-free era

The second single biggest step in the history of inguinal hernia surgery came when Theodore Billroth's dream came true. In the XIX-th century Billroth stated that: „If we could artificially produce tissues of the density and toughness of fascia and tendon, the secret of radical cure radical cure of hernia would be discovered." If Bassini idea was to reconstruct completely the inguinal canal, it was the availability of modern prosthetic materials that let perform this reconstruction in a best possible way.

The introduction of first artificial materials that could be used to reinforce herniary defect date back to 1944 when nylon has been introduced. Although the first experiences were not very promising in the years to come several new materials have been patented and become commercially available: in 1958 polietylene, in 1959 politetrafluoroetilene (PTFE) and in 1963 goretex.

Apart from many small details that differentiate various tension-free (i.e.: with some kind of mesh implant) techniques the fundamental is the position of the mesh. In general the terms „onlay" and „sublay" were in reference to the position of mesh in relation to posterior wall of the inguinal canal. The „onlay" technique (Figure 5) consist on placing the mesh superficially to posterior inguinal canal wall and „sublay" position requires formation of space for mesh in the preperitoneal space (Figure 6 and Figure 7). The more popular „onlay" techniques include the modifications by: Lichtenstein, Gilbert, Rutkow-Robbins, Trabucco, Valenti as well as PHS-Prolene Hernia System method.

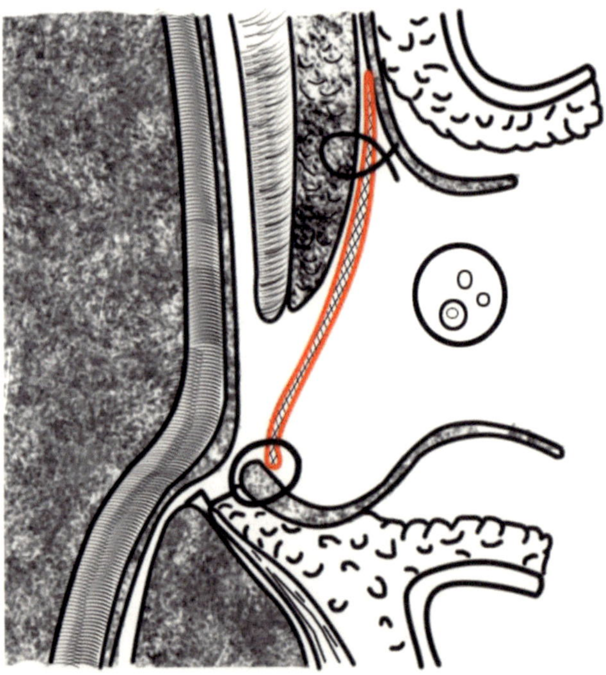

Figure 5. The "onlay" position of the mesh (in red); here in the Lichtenstein repair. Drawing by dr Jerzy W.Mituś based on Gangeri G. Risorse in chirurgia generale. Kofler Editore, Bassano del Grappa 2006 [12].

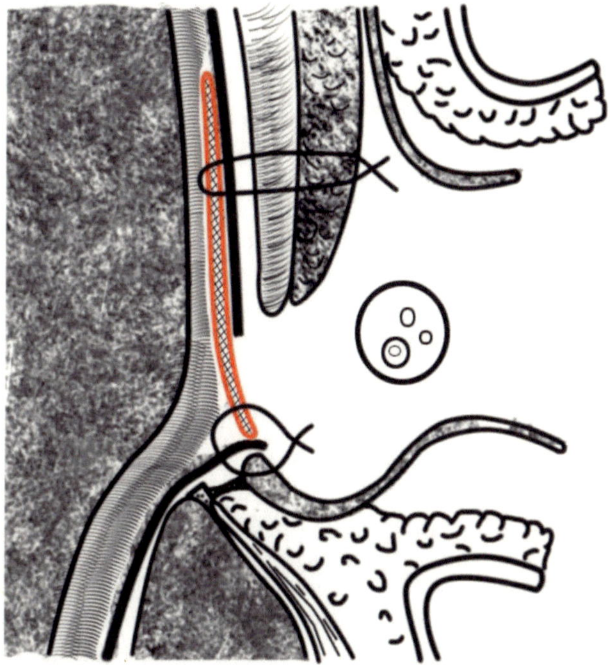

Figure 6. The "sublay" position of the mesh (in red). Drawing by dr Jerzy W.Mituś based on Gangeri G. Risorse in chirurgia generale. Kofler Editore, Bassano del Grappa 2006 [12].

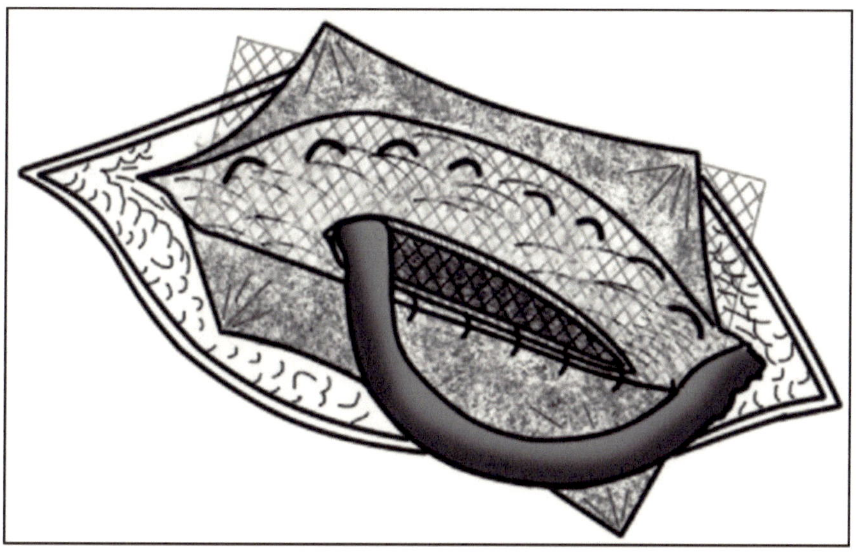

Figure 7. The "sublay" position of the mesh as seen upfront. Drawing by dr Jerzy W.Mituś based on Gangeri G. Risorse in chirurgia generale. Kofler Editore, Bassano del Grappa 2006 [12].

Initially the idea was to use the mesh to reinforce the posterior wall of the inguinal canal after performing a standard repair as in „tense" repairs. For example in the technique described in 1959 by Francis Usher the defect was reconstruct as in the Bassini operation and the Marlex (polietilene) mesh was placed on the reconstructed posterior wall to reinforce the approximated tissues [18].

It wasn't until 1984 when Irvin Lichtenstein from Los Angeles proposed repairing the posterior wall of inguinal canal with mesh without previous incision and reconstruction. In his own words: „There is evidence that to incise a strong posterior layer and, then, to reconstruct it as in the Bassini, Shouldice or McVay repair is inappropriate, disruptive and even meddlesome. The application of a wide sheet of harmless prosthetic mesh, one which serves only to strengthen such a floor, is harmless and should reduce the incidence of recurrences" [19]. And indeed the results of Lichtenstein repair were excellent: in a first 1000 patients operated by Lichtenstein and followed 5 years after surgery there weren't a single case of recurrence. It was truly a remarkable result and this is clearly one of the reasons the Lichtenstein repair is popular until today.

It was also Lichtenstein who introduce the concept of „cigarette" plug made from marlex mesh to repair fenmoral defect. This concept has been further developed by Arthur Gilbert from Miami who proposed preparing a cone from mesh and introduce it through the herniary defect without the use of sutures. This technique finally developed further when Ira Rutkow and Alan Robins from New Jersey described repair with both mesh (as in Lichtenstein repair) and plug (as in Gilbert technique). At first the technique coined „plugstein" was performed without sutures to finally reach a phase with the use of fixating sutures [20].

More recently in 1999 Arthur Gilbert described a technique that allows to place a mesh both in „onlay" and „sublay" position. His Prolene Hernia System (PHS) consisted on introducing a sophisticated mesh build from two meshes of different shape connected with a small tube. This allowed to reinforce the posterior wall of the inguinal canal both from preperitoneal site and from the „onlay" position [21]. In Table 2 the most important steps in tension-free repair can be observed.

Author	Year	Technique
Francis Usher	1959	reinforcing Bassini technique with mesh
Irvin Lichtenstein	1984	placing the mesh to reinforce the posterior wall of the inguinal canal
Arthur Gilbert	1987	cone-plug to cover defect
Ira Rutkow and Alan Robins	1998	mesh and plug repair
Arthur Gilbert	1999	Prolene Hernia System

Table 2. Techniques in tension-free repairs

http://dx.doi.org/10.5772/58533

4. Preperitoneal repair

In 1969 Rene Stoppa from Amiens developed a technique of GPRVS (giant prosthetic reinforcement of the visceral sac). This technique was supposed to be applied to large, complicated and bilateral inguinal hernias and consisted on implanting a large polyester mesh in preperitoneal connective tissue between the peritoneum and *fascia transversalis*. The incision of choice for preperitoneal access was a low midline incision and the mesh need not to be fixed with sutures due to its size and intraabdominal pressure maintaining it in situ [22]. Another preperitoneal hernia repair was described in 1976 by Lloyd Nyhus from Chicago. Unlike in the Stoppa method the incision was made above the inguinal ligament. A similar incision was used also for a preperitoneal placement of a sutureless mesh by Robert Kugel from Olimipia in his technique described in 1999 and coined Kugel Hernia Patch [23].

5. Laparoscopic hernia operations

The advent of minimally invasive techniques have seen an important number of laparoscopic and endoscopic approaches to inguinal hernia. A TAPP (transabdominal pre-peritoneal) technique described in 1993 is based on the same principle as the technique published by Lawson Tait in 1891. Tait described a transabdominal approach to inguinal hernia performed simultaneously with other interventions requiring a laparotomy [24]. In TAPP the same rationale is used in laparoscopy and an artificial mesh is placed in preperitoneal position after incising the peritoneum [25]. Another endoscopic procedure is TEP (totally extraperitoneal) in which an endoscope is introduced into Retzius and Bogros space after creating a space for gas insuflation with a specially designed balloon [26]. Afterwards, a mesh is placed in preperitoneal space and the operation is concluded. And finally an IPOM (intraperitoneal onlay mesh) is a laparoscopic technique developped in 1991 and consisting on placing a politetrafluoretilene mesh directly on the defect from pertitoneal side and securing it with a double crown of staplers [27].

After initial enthusiasm for the endoscopic hernia repairs it became clear that although these techniques have some important advantages for patients in no way can they be considered the ideal operation for every patient. Today, endoscopic techniques, while still popular in some centers, coexist peacefully with traditional open techniques of hernia repair. In a review of inguinal hernia repairs performed in USA until 2003 the most commonly used techniques were: Lichtenstein repair (350.000/year), Rutkow-Robins repair (200.000/year), endoscopic repairs (75.000/year), Bassini repair (50.000/year), McVay (less than 50.000/year) and Shouldice repair (less than 50.000/year) [28]. The use of endoscopic techniques is commonly accepted for the treatment of recurrent and bilateral hernias. As seen in the numbers cited above, when facing a non-complicated primary inguinal hernia the vast majority of today's surgeons choose tension-free repairs as described by Lichtenstein and Rutkow [29].

6. Conclusion

The surgical treatment of inguinal hernia has made important steps forward during the last 125 years. However, the fact that we still employ a wide variety of techniques to operate on inguinal hernia clearly shows that the road to a perfect operation is still ahead of us.

Acknowledgements

The author wish to thank dr Jerzy W.Mituś from Kraków, Poland for the preparation of the Figures 4, 5, 6 and 7.

Author details

Andrzej L. Komorowski

Department of Surgical Oncology, Maria Skłodowska-Curie Memorial Cancer Centre, Kraków, Poland

References

[1] Cosmacini G. La vita nelle mani. Storia della chirurgia. Gius.Laterza & Figli,Roma-Bari 2003.

[2] Sachs M, Damm M, Encke A. Historical evolution of inguinal hernia repair. World J Surg 1997;21:218-223

[3] Komorowski AL, Moran Rodriguez J. Amyand's hernia. Historical perspective and current considerations. Acta Chir Belg. 2009 Jul-Aug;109(4):563-4

[4] Tatay FC. Aproximacion historica al conocimiento de la hernia. Los medicos que la describieron y trataron. Hernia inguinocrural. Ethicon, Valencia 2001.

[5] Thomas AD, Rogers A. Edoardo Bassini and the Wound That Inspires. World Journal of Surgery 2004,28:1060–1062.

[6] Czerny V. Studien zur radikalbehandlung der hernien. Wiener Medizinische Wochenschrift 1877, 27: 497.

[7] Wood J. On rupture, inguinal, crural, and umbilical; the anatomy, pathology, diagnosis, cause, and prevention, with new methods of effecting a radical and permanent cure, embodying the Jacksonian prize essay of the Royal College of Surgeons. Davies, London 1863

[8] Legutko J, Pach R, Solecki R, Matyja A, Kulig J. The history of treatment of groin hernia. Folia Med Cracov. 2008;49(1-2):57-74.

[9] Bassini E. Sulla cura radicale dell'hernia inguinale. Archivio della societ. italiana di chirurgia 1887,4:380.

[10] Bassini E. Ueber de Bechandlung des Leistenbruches. Archiv fu®r Klinische Chirurgie 1894, 40: 429–476.

[11] Catterina A. L'operazione di Bassini per la cura radicale dell'hernia inguinale. L.Capelli, Bolonia 1932.

[12] Halsted W. The radical cure of hernia. Bull Johs Hopkins Hosp 1889;1:12

[13] Gangeri G. Risorse in chirurgia generale. Kofler Editore, Bassano del Grappa 2006.

[14] Sławiński Z. Uproszczony sposb operowania przepukliny pachwinowej. Pamiętniki Towarzystwa Lekarskiego Warszawskiego 1916, 112: 206.

[15] McVay CB. A fundamental error in current methods of inguinal herniorraphy. Surg Gynecol Obstet 1942 ;74:746

[16] Bendavid R. The Shouldice technique: a canon in hernia repair. Can J Surg. 1997 Jun; 40(3):199-205, 207

[17] Bossotti M, Balcet F, Martino F, Manfredi S, Vasario U. Inguinal hernia: technics compared in our experience. Hernioplasties compared. Minerva Chir. 1994;49(12): 1269-73.

[18] Usher F. Hernia repair with Marlex mesh. An analysis of 541 cases. Arch Surg 1962;84:73

[19] Lichtenstein IL, Shulman AG. Ambulatory (outpatient) hernia surgery including a new concept: introducing tension-free repair. Int Surg 1986;71:1

[20] Rutkow IM, Robbins AW. The Marlex mesh PerFix groin hernioplasty. Europ J Surg 1998:164:549

[21] Gilbert AI. Underlay-onlay mesh hernia device: initial report. Hernia 1999:3;4

[22] Stoppa R, Quintyn M. Les deficiences de la paroi abdominale chez le subject age: colloque avec le practicien. Sem Hosp 1969;45:2182

[23] Kugel RD. Minimally invasive, non laparoscopic, preperitoneal, and sutureless, inguinal herniorraphy. Am J Surg 1999;178:298

[24] Tait L. A discussion on treatment of hernia by median abdominal section. Br Med J 1891;34:685

[25] Litwin DE, Pham QN, Oleniuk FH, Kluftinger AM, Rossi L. Laparoscopic groin hernia surgery: the TAPP procedure. Transabdominal preperitoneal hernia repair. Can J Surg. 1997 Jun;40(3):192-8

[26] McKernan JB, Laws HL. Laparoscopic repair of inguinal hernias using a totally extraperitoneal prosthetic approach. Surg Endosc. 1993 Jan-Feb;7(1):26-8

[27] Toy FK, Smoot RT Jr. Toy-Smooth laparoscopic hernioplasty. Surg Laparosc Endosc. 1991 Sep;1(3):151-5

[28] Rutkow IM. Demographic and socioeconomic aspects of hernia repair in the United States in 2003. Surg Clin North Am. 2003 Oct;83(5):1045-51, v-vi.

[29] Nathan JD, Pappas TN. Inguinal hernia: an old condition with new solutions. Ann Surg. 2003;238(6 Suppl):S148-57.

Section 2

Laparoscopic Treatment

Chapter 2

Groin Hernia Repair in Laparoscopic Era

Süleyman Çetinkünar, Hasan Erdem,
B. Çağlar Bilgin, Seyfi Emir, İlhan Bali and
Selim Sözen

Additional information is available at the end of the chapter

http://dx.doi.org/10.5772/57250

1. Introduction

Inguinal hernias are a common pathology. The use of a non-absorbable mesh placed in the preperitoneal space for the treatment of inguinal hernias was first introduced by Rives in 1966 [1]. Stoppa introduced the use of a large mesh prosthesis via a posterior approach for the repair of bilateral hernias [2]. Open and endoscopic procedures have been described for hernia surgery since Bassini in 1887 [3] Inguinal hernia treatment offers many possibilities, such as the laparoscopic approach, of which several techniques have been described. Ever since its initial definition in 1990, laparoscopic inguinal hernia repair has gained significant progress [4]. Laparoscopic inguinal hernia repair was first performed using the transabdominal approach, wherein the intra-peritoneal techniques, such as onlay or plug mesh application on the upper ligation of the peritoneum, were employed. Upon observation of early recurrence, the practice of placing the mesh between the peritoneum and the muscle directly led to the emergence of the TAPP and TEP techniques. Only these two laparoscopic repairs have proven to be viable, with early results comparable or superior to the Liechtenstein repair. In brief, the TAPP method involves entering the abdomen with trocars, opening the peritoneum in the hernia zone, covering the potential hernia zones with the mesh and then re-suturing the opened peritoneum. The primary superiority of the TAPP technique versus the TEP technique is that it has an early learning curve. The TEP technique does not involve entering the peritoneal cavity but rather restricts the work to only the Retzius' space. It enables the placement of a large preperitoneal mesh, with the several advantages including the repair of bilateral hernias, minimal dissection, elimination of performing a pneumoperitoneum and addressing its attendant complications, quick return to normal activity after repair, cosmesis and excellent long-term results. In comparison to open surgery methods, endoscopic hernia repair, using either TAPP or TEP procedures, involves less pain and minimal recurrent rates.

2. Anatomy

The early 1900s serves as an important period in the development of inguinal hernia surgery. During this period, cadaveric and clinical studies were able to better explain the anatomy of the inguinal canal. Many topics that had not been properly understood and therefore unable to be adequately investigated had begun to be illuminated with the anatomy atlases and new books by Astley Cooper [5], Franz Hasselbach [6], Antonia Scarpa, Jules Germain Cloquet [7] and Morton [8]. The significance of the rear wall of the inguinal canal in etiology and the repair of inguinal hernias was more clearly understood as a result of this new knowledge. It has been revealed that the defect in transverse muscle aponeurosis and transverse fascia plays an important role in the emergance of hernias. The objective in the rectification of this defect is to prevent tension in the transverse fascia [5,8,9].

3. Inguinal canal

In an adult, the inguinal canal is an approximately 4 cm - length oblique path at the bottom of the anterior abdominal wall. It is situated between the external (superficial) and internal (profound) inguinal rings at 2-4 cm above the top of the inguinal ligament [10], (Figure 1, 3). Hernia repairs performed using the anterior approach begin with an oblique incision of the external ring and continues to the anteromedial aspect of the cord at the level of the internal ring, proceeding then to the search for an indirect hernia sac at the level of the internal ring at the anteromedial aspect of the cord [13].

External Ring: The triangle-shaped aperture of the external oblique aponeurosis created by its base, whose superior and inferior legs are limited by the upper part of the pubic bone. While the superior leg is formed by external oblique aponeurosis itself, the inferior leg is formed by the inguinal ligament [7,14]. The superior leg is attached to the lateral border of rectus sheath and the tendon of rectus abdominis muscle sheath, and the inferior leg is attached to the pubic tubercle.

Internal Ring: A U-shaped normal aperture in the transverse fascia. The boundaries of this reverse U is formed by the front and rear transverse fascia. Its lower limit is formed by the illiobic tract of the specialized thickening of the transverse fascia [7,14], (Figure 1). Henri Fruchaud (1894 - 1960) was an anatomist surgeon who gathered all inguinal hernias under a single etiology and ushered in the concept of "Myopectineal Aperture" to hernia anatomy. Fruchaud categorized the hernias according to their clinical presentations and believed that they began from the place himself was responsible for defining as the myopectineal orifice. The boundaries of this space are constituted by the upper internal oblique muscle fibers, the transversus abdominis muscle, the outer iliopsoas muscle, the inner rectus muscle's lateral limit and the bottom pecten pubis. The inguinal ligament passes over this structure and ramifies into two. The spermatic cord and femoral veins pass through this area. It is internally covered by the transverse fascia only [9,10], (Figure-4).

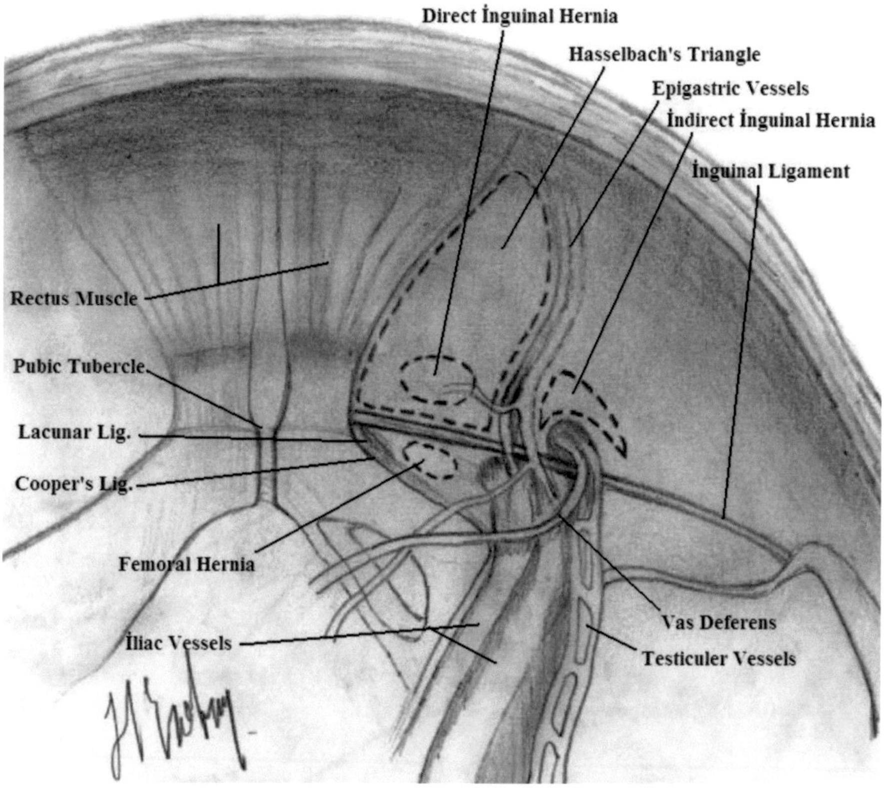

Figure 1. Posterior anatomy of inguinal region

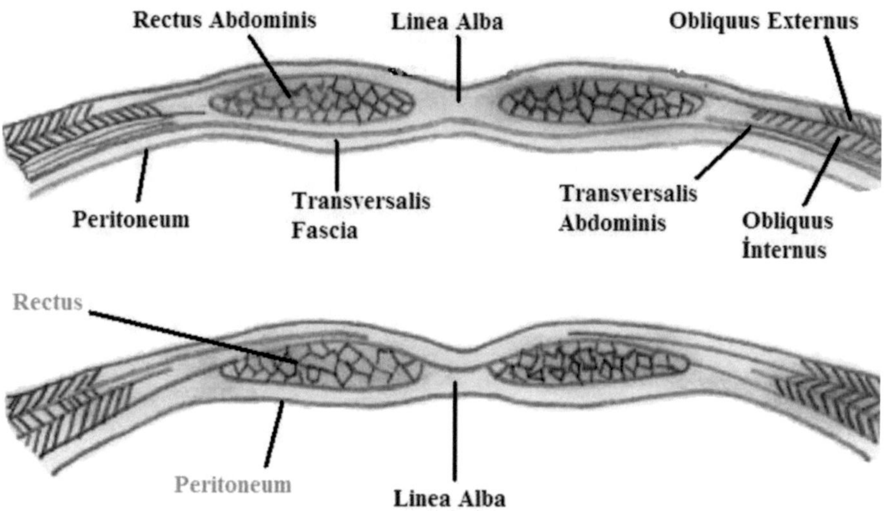

Figure 2. Anterior and lateral abdominal wall layers

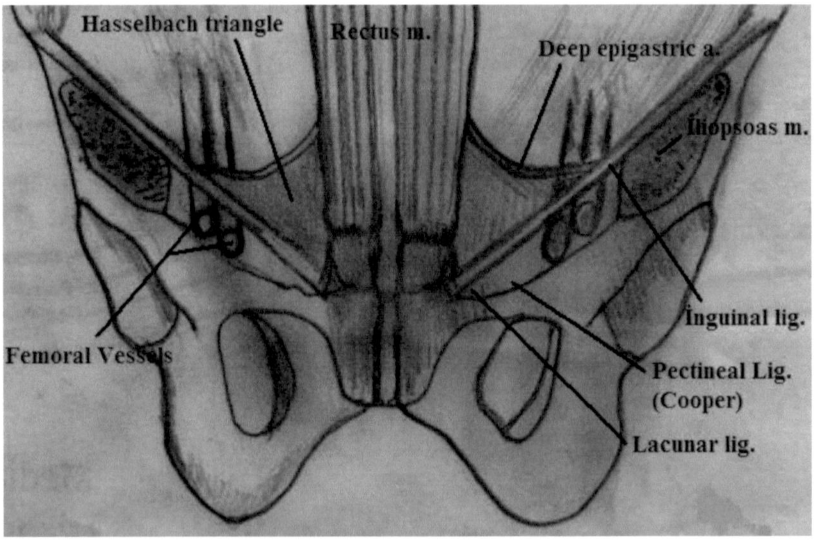

Figure 3. Ligaments of inguinal region

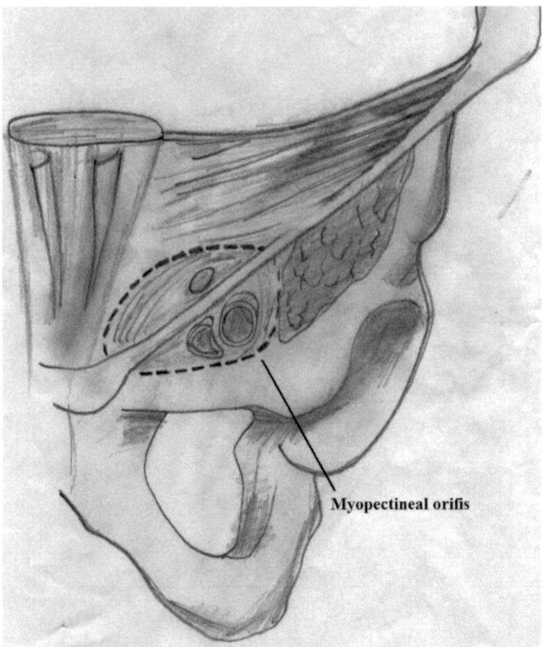

Figure 4. Myopectineal Orifice of Fruchaud

Hasselbach's Triangle:

The lateral border of the superior or inferior Hasselbach triangle is formed by the inferior epigastric vessels, the medial border by the lateral rectus abdominis muscle and the inferolateral border by the inguinal ligament. Most of the direct hernias and external supravesicle inguinal hernias emanate from here [10,15], (Figure 2).

Cooper Ligament (Ligamentum pectineale):

This ligament starts from the pubic tubercle and continues along the linea pectinea. It disappears by becoming thinner adjacent to eminentia iliopectinea. It has a 30-degree angular difference with the Poupart ligament and is a strong structure [10,13,15], (Figure 1).

Anatomy of the posterior inguinal region:

When viewed from the abdominal to suprapubic and inguinal area, three peritoneal folds and three shallow fossas extending downward from the omphaloe are seen.

Plica Umbilicalis Mediana:

The part of the urachus that extends from the omphaloe to the bladder. It is located beneath the linea alba and is quite hard to discern (it can be more distinct in some people).

Plica Umbilicalis Medialis:

Remnants of the umbilical artery extending from the omphaloe down to the iliac arteries. They are located in the medial position of the epigastric vessels. Because they serve no function in the human body, incisions made on them do not cause any harm.

Plica Umbilicalis Lateralis:

It is created by the epigastric artery and vein and requires attention when performing dissection.

Lateral fossa:

It is limited by the medial inferior epigastric artery. An internal inguinal ring (indirect inguinal hernia outlet) is present in it.

Medial fossa:

It is found between the inferior epigastric artery and the medial umbilical ligament (remnant of the umbilical artery). Direct inguinal hernias protrude out of it.

Supravesical fossa:

It is situated between medial and the median umbilical ligaments (Median umbilical ligament: Umbilical artery remnants). Supravesicle external hernias protrude from here [10,12], (Figure 5).

Arteria Epigastrica İinferior:

It is a branch of A. Iliaca externa. Advancing through rear peritoneal and transverse fascia, it crosses iliopubic tract and reaches the level of medial edge of inner ring and extends inwardly and upwardly. At the level of linea semicircular, it makes an anastomosis with A. Epigastrica superior. It feeds the rectus muscle.

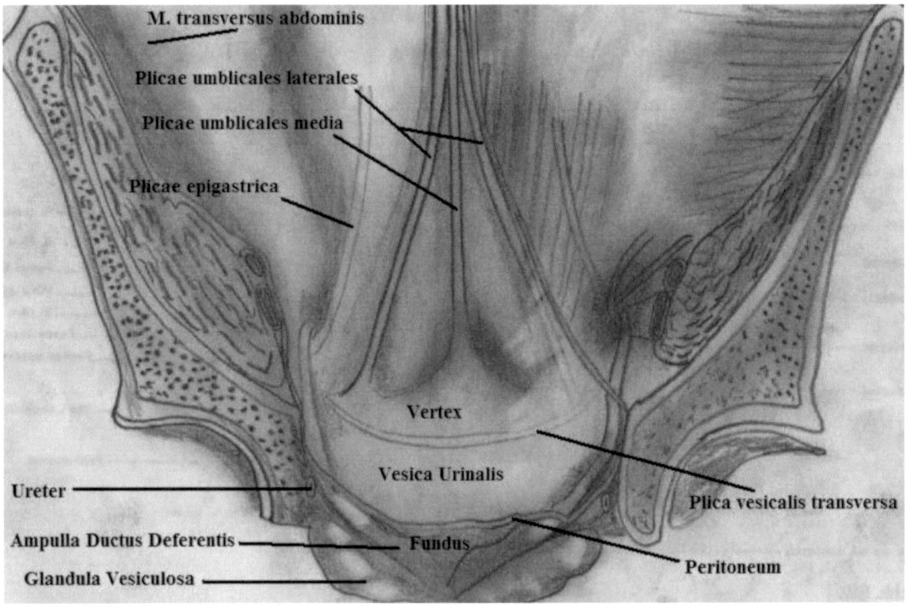

Figure 5. Preperitoneal view of lower abdomen

In the endoscopic repair of groin hernia, when the peritoneum is left at posterior and viewed from the anterior abdominal wall, 2 rectus abdominis muscles vertically extend from pubis at the centerline of anterior abdominal wall towards thoracic cage.

Anterior abdominal wall: It is composed of two sections (Figure 2):

Medial Section	Lateral Section
M.Rectus Abdominis	M.Obliquus Externus Abdominis
M.Piramidalis	M. Obliquus Internus Abdominis
	M.Transversus Abdominis
	M.Cremastericus

The medial section of anterior abdominal wall is formed by the rectus abdominis and pyramidal muscles. The rectus muscles on both sides are traversed by three tendinous lines. These traversing points occur at the level of xiphoid projection and omphaloe in such a way so as to stay in the middle of these two. These tendinous bands are tightly attached to the front fold of the rectus sheath (7).

Rectus muscle is firmly closed with the bilaminar aponeuroses formed by three superficial anterior and exterior muscles. It is formed by the exterior sheath, transversus abdominis, transverse posterior fold of internal oblique aponeurosis, of the transversus abdominis aponeurosis and transverse fascia until a distance from the rib border is reached so as to align with the center section of the omphaloe and pubic (linea semicircular). Exterior sheath beneath this point is developed solely by the transverse fascia [7,12]. Lateral abdominal wall consists of three layers of muscle: External oblique, internal oblique and transversus abdominis muscles.

Each is wrapped with a separate fascia and terminates at the bottom as a flat tendon or aponeurosis returns. The outermost external oblique muscle that starts on the posterior part of the lower eight ribs and descends downward in a wrapping manner around the body. This muscle, which continues up to a line drawn from the anterior superior of the iliac spine to the umbilicusas, turns into aponeurosis below this limit and envelops the ilioinguinal region beneath the innominate fascia. The lacunare ligament, inguinal ligament and the inguinal ligament reflexum are structures related to the aponeurosis. The inguinal ligament (Poupart) forms the outer edge of the oblique aponeurosis and extends from the anterior superior iliac spine towards the tubercle pubicum. From the termination point of the Poupart ligament, a band called the Lacunar ligament (Gimbernard ligamant) extends towards the pubis. A triangle-shaped formation that is 1.25 cm in length. The fibers of the external oblique aponeurosis just above the inguinal ligament and at the lateral of its bonding location inside the pubic tubercle branches out to construct an aperture, which functions as the exterior (superficial) inguinal ring. The spermatic cord passes through the aperture in males and the round ligament in females [10,12].

The internal oblique muscle begins at the half-way point of the lateral ligament and adjacent iliac fascia and at the 2/3 point of the anterior iliac crest and lower parts of the adjacent lumbar aponeurosis.

The aponeurosis of this muscle extends towards the medial and makes up the anterior rectus sheath uniting with the aponeurosis of the transversus abdominis muscle beneath the semicircular line. The bottom fibers of the muscle make up the cremasteric muscle adhering to the spermatic cord [12].

The transversus abdominis muscle is the deepest muscle layer in this region. The lateral part of the iliopubic tract of the inner part of the iliac crest starts from the inner surface of lumbodorsal fascia and lower six ribs' cartilage. It transversely passes through abdominal side wall towards medial. The muscle fibers then transform into tendinous aponeurosis at the rectus sheath uniting with the internal oblique aponeurosis. The transversus abdominis muscle creates a free edge by twisting over its free bottom part and internal inguinal ring. This is called the aponeurotic arch of the posterior transversus abdominis and generally combines with the internal oblique aponeurosis nearby the spot where it adheres to the pubic tubercle, and it forms the "Joint" (conjoint) tendon. It is seen in only 5% of the humans and is the basic structure utilized in the anatomic repair.

3.1. Bogros space

Fatty and other connective tissues are situated on the left aperture between the peritoneum, also referred to as the Bogros space, and the posterior fold of the transverse fascia. Today, the Bogros space, which was defined by a French surgeon in 1823, does not receive full acceptance in terms of the anatomic structures it contains. However, what matters is that it has become the space where the synthetic prostheses are today placed in modern hernia surgery [11,12,18].

According to Bendavid, the Bogros space is the lateral extension of the retropubic zone of the Retzius' Space. The Bogros space can be exposed by making an incision from the tranverse fascia of the inner ring down to the pubic bone. A venous plexus is present at the bottom and anterior sections of the Bogros space. Bendavid's venous circle is found at the subinguinal section of the Bogros space and is comprised of the following structures: Deep inferior epigastric vein, iliopubic vein, rectal veins the retropubic vein and the unifying rectus epigastric vein [18].

3.2. Inguinal nerve region

Iliohypogastric, ilioinguinal nerves and the genital branch of the genitofemoral nerve are of primary importance for the surgeon presiding over the operation. The iliohypogastric and ilioinguinal nerves unifying and advancing their routes in approximately 25% of the cases provide the sensory innervation of the skin of the inguinal zone, the base of the penis and the anterior side of the upper abdominal region. The position of these nerves protruding from T12-L1 is variable. Its existence above the spermatic cord, which is the typical localization of the ilioinguinal nerve, is encountered in only 60% of the cases. In addition, it might be found in or behind the the cremaster muscle.

As for the genital nerve, it contains both motor and sensory fibers. It innervates the cremaster muscle, lateral skin of scrotum and the labia, stemming up from L1-2. It is situated across the iliopubic tract inside the inguinal canal [10,16].

3.3. Spermatic cord structures

The spermatic cord (funiculus spermaticus) emerges from the preperitoneal space at the level of the anterior ring and comes out of the outer ring after passing through inguinal canal and upper lateral section of pubis and combines with the testicle in the scrotum.

In the spermatic nerve functioning as a branch of the genitofemoral nerve that accommodates the adipose tissue and lymphatics, spermatic artery, plexus pampiniformis and ductus deferens are present. The plexus pampiniformis ensures drainage of spermatic cord veins and forms the testicular vein at the level of the anterior ring. Similarly, a peritoneal fold is present inside the cord. Initially, this structure is in the form of a sac (processus vaginalis), but at a later point closes. The layers making up the cord from inside to outward order: 1 - Internal spermatic fascia: The continuation of transverse fascia encircling the cord up to testicle. 2 - The middle layer (Cremaster muscle): The continuation of internal oblique muscle. It provides roots up to the testicles. 3 - External spermatic fascia: The continuation of aponeurosis of the external oblique fascia (Fascia nominata of Gallaudet fascia) encircling the cord up to testicle [5,9,11].

4. Indications

The general indications for laparoscopic inguinal hernia repair, TAPP or TEP are the same as they are for open inguinal hernia repair. For young, active males with primary hernias, it may

http://dx.doi.org/10.5772/57250

ofter decreased pain and an earlier return to activity. Laparoscopy may be ideal for bilateral groin hernias and recurrences from open approaches, but is also appropriate with unilateral primary hernias when the surgeon and patient are comfortable with the procedure.

Laparoscopic groin hernia classification is closely related to Nyhus [19], with all the anatomical aspects described according to this procedure

Type 1: Congenital hernias with a narrow internal ring

Type 2 : External oblique inguinal hernias with a dilated internal ring

Type 3:

a. The posterior wall of the inguinal canal is damaged

b. External oblique hernias with a dilated internal ring.

c. Femoral hernias identified in the medial inguinal region below the inguinal ligament

Type 4: Recurrent hernias

The laparoscopic procedure can be considered for all adult patients, regardless of the type of hernia. The best indications according to this classification are;

- Type 3 hernias
- Bilateral hernias
- Type 4 hernias,

Obesity, strenuous activities (strenuous working and sports).

Relative indications:

- Type I or II hernias except when associated with another type of hernia or in cases of bilateral hernias; voluminous sliding hernias;
- strangulated hernias, diagnosed early.

5. Contraindications

There are very few contraindications for these procedures. Some of them are listed below;

- contraindication to general anesthesia;
- extensive intra-abdominal adhesions;
- extremely voluminous sliding hernias with the bowel attached to the hernia sac;
- late diagnosis of strangulated hernias with advanced bowel obstruction.

Prior lower abdominal surgery or pelvic radiation are strong relative contraindications.

6. Surgical technique

6.1. Equipment used in laparoscopic repair

Insufflation needle (Veress: Palmer): In the intra-abdominal approaches, it is required for CO2 insufflation into abdominal cavity. For the intra-abdominal pressure, 12mmHg is adequate. Since entry is made through the use of trocars; there is no need for any insufflation needles, such as Veress, in the total extraperitoneal method. Maintaining the cavity formed by this method at 8 - 10 mmHg with CO2 pressure is adequate.

Trocars: Generally, three trocar entries are sufficient for laparoscopic repair. In almost all repair techniques, a 10-mm trocar is applied just below the umbilicus for the telescope input and the input for the balloon trocars. Specially designed balloon trocars are used for the TEP technique. By virtue of these trocars, entry into the Retzius' space from the umbilical zone and the creation of a potential cavity inside the preperitoneal area is greatly facilitated (Figure 6).

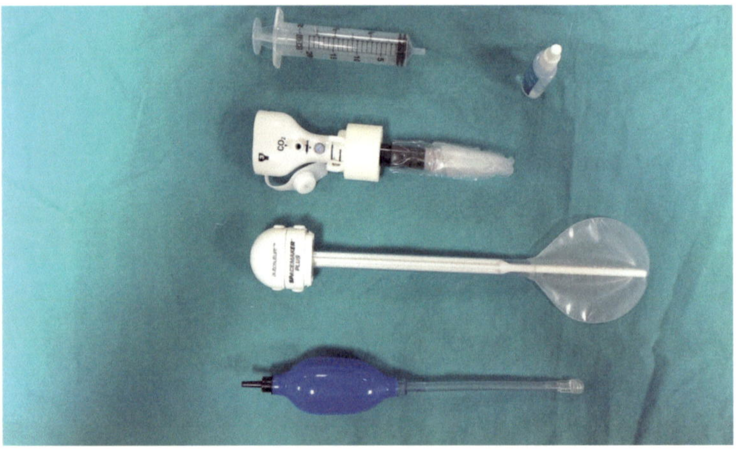

Figure 6. Baloon Trocars (from Çetinkünar's archive)

Telescope: While a standard telescope can be employed, the use of a 30-degree angular telescope ensures large-scaled visibility.

Manipulation Equipment

1. Grasper and Dissector: Both grasper and dissectors can be used with 5mm trocars.
2. Electrocautery and Scissors: Use of electrocautery in the inguinal region where the great vessels are situated when applying the transabdominal preperitoneal procedure and total extraperitoneal method requires that great care be taken.
3. Aspiration - Irrigation Equipment: These can be used both for stopping hemorrhages which could potentially occur during dissection and for the purpose of cleaning the area as well. However, since frequent aspiration and irrigation might disturb the camera image, use of small buffers is also recommended.

4. Endoclip: For controlling the hemorrhages which might occur, the endoclip must be available among the tools to be used. Particularly, injury to the inferior epigastric veins passing right through the middle of the dissection area may require it to be ligated with the endoclip.

5. Endo-Stitch: An apparatus facilitating placement of suture in closure of peritoneal or hernia sac (TAPP procedure).

6. Endo peanut: Used for the blunt dissection.

7. Mesh stabilizer: Available in absorbable and non-absorbable, anchor and helical types and are effective in the fixed attachment of the prosthesis at appropriate locations. In some selected cases fibrin glue or sealant may be used.

6.2. Prostheses

Laparoscopic hernia repair techniques require the use of a prosthesis. The use of a prosthesis provides advantages such as low rates of recurrence and the prevention of tension. The polypropylene mesh produced for this purpose in non-absorbable and monofilament form is currently the most effective and commonly applied prosthesis material. In the repair of hernias, different raw materials and types of mesh can be used, such as anatomically shaped meshes(Figure 7). The properties to look for in meshes are as follows:

- Monofilament, pore size greater than 10 μm
- Easy transformability into the shape of the space it is placed
- Resistance to adhesion or erosion of organs
- Anti-allergic and protection against foreign body reaction
- Infection resistance
- Ability to withstand physiological stress for adequate time

Preparing the patient for surgery: Prior to the operation, it is required that patient be informed of the benefits of the laparoscopic repair of inguinal hernia, its potential risks and the availability of the open surgery option. The patient's consent should be obtained in writing. Since the use of mesh will be necessary for skin flora suppression, first-generation cephalosporins are administered parenteral. Patients are asked to urinate on the morning of surgery. For those patients who are unable to do so, a bladder catheter may be applied on the operating table. This is important for not to damage bladder during surgery.

Patient position:

The patient is laid in supine position with arms fastened. Following general anesthesia, the operating table is brought to 20 degrees - Trendelenburg position and the patient is rotated by 25-30 degrees in adverse direction of the side where the hernia repair would be actualized (sided, tilted). Thus, blockage of view by the intraperitoneal organs may be prevented at the

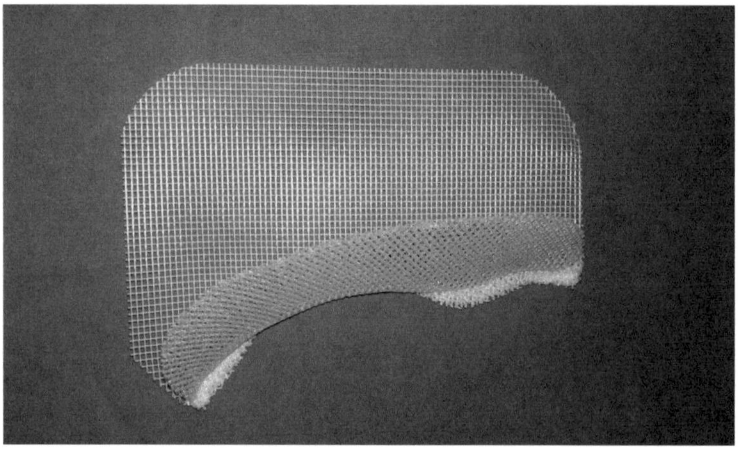

Figure 7. Anatomical shaped mesh for TEP (from Çetinkünar's archive)

repair area during operation. As for the laparoscopy unit is placed at the toe side on the same side where hernia operation would perform

Surgery Team:

The surgeon stands on the opposite side of the zone to be repaired. Nurse and the physician stand on the same side and the assistant stands on the opposite side.

6.2.1. TAPP technique

Insertion of trocars

After having made up pre-peritoneal with Veress needle, maintaining the intra-abdominal pressure at 12 mmHg is sufficient. A 10mm trocar is inserted - depending on the preference of the surgeon either being open or closed - into abdomen for the camera just beneath the umbilicus upon an incision made. Both pubic areas should be examined for any other possible intra-abdominal pathology after carrying out exploration with the laparoscope. The trocars to be used by the surgeon and the assistant should be inserted from approximately 5 mm distance from the outer edges of rectus abdominuses in a way to be on the transverse line of umbilicus. The diameter of the trocar to be used by the surgeon must be 12 mm. A 5 - mm diameter for the third trocar and to stay on the hernia side is adequate.

Dissection of Hernia Area: Before beginning the dissection, centerline (lig.umblicale medianum) and cord elements and residential area of the hernia which can be chosen just behind the peritoneum to lig.umblicale lateral formed by medial umbilical ligament, inferior epigastric artery and vein make up the boundaries required to be recognized. Excluding some of indirect hernias, the hernia sac can be easily reversed in form of a finger of gloves by being gripped from its tip.

The dissection is commenced with a peritoneal incision so as to be approximately 1 cm above the defect extending from umbilical medial ligament up to the anterior superior of iliac spine.

This dissection can be easily done a pair of scissors with cautery or Hook. Entering the preperitoneal region, the flaps are prepared by blunt dissection up and down. The hernia sac stays at the subperitoneal flap. Although this operation is easy with direct hernia, with the cases with indirect hernia exhibiting adhesion to the spermatic cord, partly sharp dissection is required. In blunt dissections carried out from the preperitoneal distance, the anatomic structures like inferior epigastric artery and vein, and the elements of the spermatic cord and iliopubic tract, Cooper's ligament, transverse aponeurotic arch and pubis should be uncovered. When the spermatic cord was dissected together with its elements from the peritoneal flap, first step of the operation is completed. Dissection in Retzius' space is performed primarily by using traction and counter-traction. Dissection is continued until Cooper's ligament and the pubic symphysis are identified and a large space is created. Retzius' space is the prevesical space between the symphysis, the bladder, and the anterior abdominal wall. It contains loose connective tissue and fat.

Placement of mesh

This stage is the selection of a prosthesis which would cover all potential hernia spaces prepared and whose anatomic formations to be used in its repair. After being wound in roller, the prosthesis should be pushed into abdomen through 10 - 12 mm trocar. Rotation of the cord is not required in this technic at all. If the spermatic cord was not rotated, the mesh can be laid on the anatomic structures and fixed.

Mesh fixation

Laparoscopic hernia repair involves the fixation of the prosthetic mesh in the preperitoneal space with staples to avoid displacement leading to recurrence. Fixation of mesh must be made to transverse aponeurotic above and outside, to pubic bone inside and to Cooper's ligament and the ilipubic tract at lower side. The point required to pay attention very much is not to use stapler on the lateral aspect of the external iliac artery and vein and the inferior edge of the lateral pubic tract. These areas are the potential navigation zones of femoral branch of n. genitofemoralis and n.cutaneus lateralis. The last point where the upper edge of prosthesis on lateral would be attached to is the medial of anterior superior of the iliac spine so as to be on top. Use of 6 or 7 staples of staplers is adequate in fixation. One each as per corner and one each to the right and left sides of inferior epigastric vessels above the transversal aponeurotic arc and one each at pubic bone and iliopubic tract at medial should be placed. Especially in femoral and direct hernias, additional fixation also to Cooper ligament is appropriate. Some authors suggest not to fix the mesh with a staple device because of a few complications such us ostetitis, chronical groin pain, nerve injury and hematomas. For this reason mesh placement without any suture or stapler seems to be another option in endoscopic hernia repair. But disadvantage of these techniques is migration of the mesh. Just at this point the use of fibrin glue or sealant will be preferable for mesh fixation. Fibrin sealing has recently evolved as a new technique for mesh fixation in endoscopic inguinal hernia repair. Fibrin sealant is a biodegradable adhesive formed by the combination of human-derived fibrinogen and thrombin activated by calcium chloride, leading to the formation of polymerized fibrin chains. After applying the fibrin sealant, it is broken down by fibrinolysis and replaced by a fibrotic layer. The fibrinogen component gives the product its tensile strength and adhesive properties, and the thrombin component promotes fibroblast proliferation [20]. The clinical use of cyanoacrylate synthetic glues as an alternative for mesh fixation in endoscopic hernia repair. [20]

Many studies in the current literature emphasis the advantages of fibrin sealant which can be safely applied in the endoscopic and open hernia surgery. [21,22] As the overall quality of reported studies remains poor, well-designed studies in the future are needed until fibrin sealing can replace mechanical stapling as a new standard for mesh fixation

Closure of periton flaps

By closing the peritoneal flaps opened at the final stage, the contact of mesh with the intra-abdominal organs must be prevented. The upper and lower peritoneal flaps are superposed with the stapler.

Endoscopic total extraperitoneal inguinal hernia repair (TEP)

TEP is different as the peritoneal cavity is not entered and mesh is used to seal the hernia from outside the thin membrane covering the organs in the abdomen. The trocar inlets present property in this method. Following application of local anesthesia to the probable entry locations, entry of first trocar is realized with a 10 - 12 mm transverse skin incision made from the lower edge of umbilicus. If this incision is made closer to the side where the hernia exists particularly with one-sided hernias, exposure becomes better. A 1 cm - incision is made on the anterior sheath of abdominis muscle and lateralizing the rectus muscle, posterior sheath is made visible. Inserting the finger between posterior sheath and the muscle, tunnel is prepared. There are two methods in creating extraperitoneal space. First one is made by advancing a 10 mm trocar placed into such tunnel and making CO2 insufflation and trocar is pushed into Retzius' space through laparoscopic trocar being a blunt-tipped probe. Second one is the Balloon trocar which is frequently used by inserting the trocar through tunnel rim and guiding it towards symphysis pubis. In single-sided hernias, the trocar cannula should be held towards the hernia side and as for the bilateral ones, it should be held in the midline. If periton is punctured at this stage, the process should be restarted only after removal of cannula and closing the muscle anterior sheath by opening the anterior sheath of opposite rectus abdominus muscle. Arrival of cannula tip at the pubis is easily understood with an external palpation. At this stage, after changing the probe of balloon trocar with the telescope, balloon is started to be inflated. With the aid of 30 - 40 pumping action, it is inflated. Later on, in order to avoid complications and cause anatomy to be clearly exposed, landmarks are determined. The one of these landmarks firstly seen is the symphysis pubis. Until Cooper ligament is seen, balloon dissection is kept on. The balloon inflated should be maintained in place averagely for 3 minutes. This process will ensure the distance formed to be permanent and small hemorrhages to be buffered. Upon having making up the working area, balloon trocar is taken out and while it is possible to enter through same inlet with classic 10 mm trocars as well, structural balloon trocars specifically produced for commercial purpose as to be used in these operations can be used. Then, the extraperitoneal space is being inflated up to an 8 - 12 mmHg pressure. When inserting other two trocars into preperitoneal inguinal cavity, there are two different applications from the aspect of inlet points. Being most - adopted one, in the first application; 5mm trocar is inserted above pubis symphysis 2-3, other 5 cm trocar through center of umbilicus and pubis line (on the same median line with both trocars). As for the second application preferred by some surgeons, 3 trocars is inserted from one point around the hernia, a little below the umbilicus horizontal line, outer edge of rectus muscle. In some patients, creation of the pneumoperitoneum may well reduce the working space and in exceptional cases lead to a conversion towards a trans-abdominal preperitoneal (TAPP) surgery

Dissection of hernia region

Dissection should be continued to medial and lateral starting from midline. An irrigation-aspiration device with a grasper and blunt tip scissors may be used for dissection. In the extraperitoneal method, anatomical structures necessary for the fixed attachment of mesh should be exposed (Figure 10), reducing the hernia sac consisting of peritoneum. The epigastric artery and vein are exposed as 2nd landmark (Figure 8). After separation with blunt dissection from the iliac vessels behind, the spermatic cord is freed from the tissue behind with the help of a dissector at the level of inguinal annulus profundus. In the case of an indirect hernia sac, it will be located in the anteromedial aspect of the spermatic cord. Testicular vessels progress in the posterolateral aspect, vas deferens (Figure 9) in the medial aspect of the hernia sac. The hernia sac captured with a grasper will be pulled forward and inward perpendicular to the axis of the cord, as testicular veins will be freed as much as possible by pulling them outward with blunt dissection (Figure 10). If the hernia sac is small, it may be left in the preperitoneal position or the distal part may be excised, connecting the endoclip with the help of an endoloop. In the case of large hernia sacs, the excess sac may be cut after being ligated with suture or endoloop. Another option is to cut the sac at the level of the inner ring and to leave the distal part in place after closing the proximal part. Particularly in indirect congenital hernias, this operation will inevitably be performed.

Placement of mesh

The first fixed attachment to be done over the Cooper ligament facilitates the proper placement of the mesh. Occasionally, obturator vessels traversing the Cooper ligament by a curve can be found in only the medial aspect of the iliac vein. Mesh fixators should be used in this area referred to as the Corona Mortis. The space that accommodates the prosthesis should be enlarged towards the anterior superior iliac spine, and the psoas muscle, along with its various nerve rami, can be adequately visualized. These nerve rami must be preserved in order to avoid post-operative neuralgia. This area is called the triangle of pain, and it is absolutely impermissible to place any fixation device in this area as this would increase the risk of stapling a nerve ramus, an error that would lead to immediate and refractory post-operative pain and necessitate a second intervention to remove the staple responsible for the pain. The fibrin glue or sealant usage in this cases may prevent these complications with similar recurrence rates.

The procedure is terminated after the mesh is placed. Withdrawal of the gas should be done slowly under direct supervision. In order to avoid folding of the upper and lower edges that couldn't be fixed, they should be properly overlaid with the help of a grasper during the withdrawal of the gas. Fascia in the 12 mm and 10 mm trocar sites are closed with absorbable suture material.

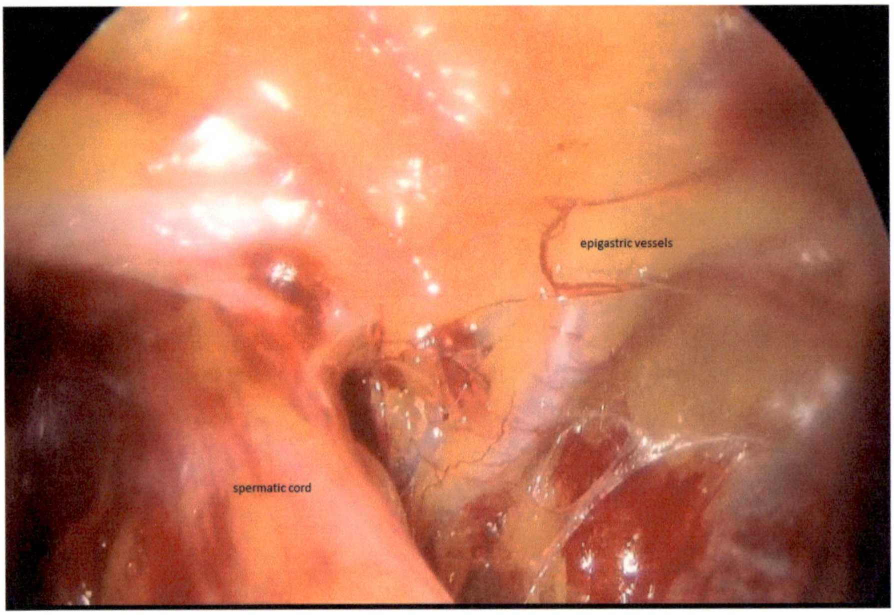

Figure 8. Inferior epigastric vessels (from Çetinkünar's archive)

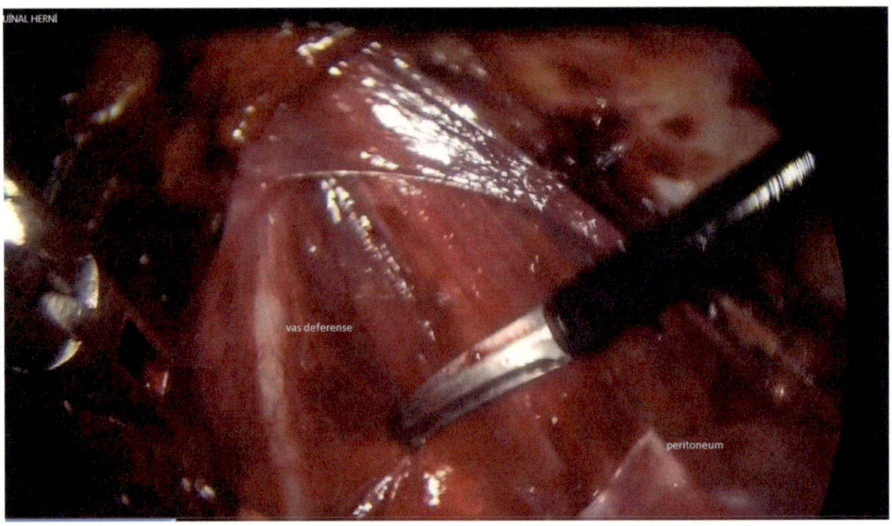

Figure 9. Vas deferense (from Çetinkünar's archive)

7. Post-operative care

On the day of surgery, the anesthetic effect wears off after 6-8 hours and then patients are mobilized and oral food intake is initiated. The patient may be discharged on the same day of surgery. In general, patients who no longer need to take analgesics after the 3rd day may go

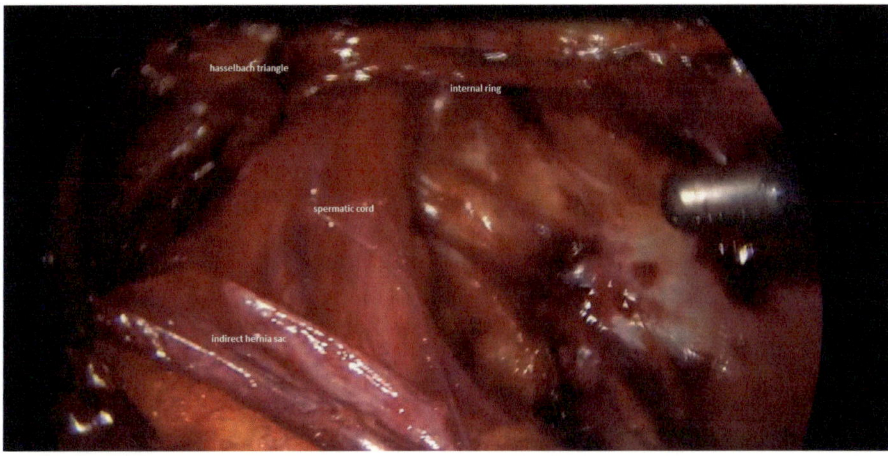

Figure 10. Hernia sac (peritoneum)dissection (from Çetinkünar's archive)

on with their normal activities. Active employees and athletes may return to full activity after two weeks.

8. Complications

The overall incidence of morbidity after laparoscopic groin hernia repair has been quite variable. Unfortunately, it will never be possible to completely eliminate complications after laparoscopic hernioplasty, but it is possible to reduce their incidence. A thorough knowledge of the anatomy and the operative approach, along with advanced laparoscopic skills will reduce the possibility of significant complications. Serious complications specific to the laparoscopic technique, although reduced in parallel with training and experience, seen especially in the early stages of hernia surgery and mostly associated with TAPP, have been reported. Complication rates vary from 3% to 25%. [23,24]. Fortunately, serious complications are uncommon. A summary of possible complications is shown in Table 1. If we take a look at the most common complications;

1. Laparoscopy related complications:

a. Vascular injuries:

The most common vascular injuries are epigastric artery vein and spermatic vein injuries. In the literature, external iliac, obturator veins and deep circumflex iliac vessel injuries have been reported. Particularly during mesh fixation, Corona Mortis injuries may also be seen. Dorsal penile vein injury has been reported as well during balloon dissections. The incidence of hemorrhage after TEP surgery is 0.4%. [25]. The rate of major vessel injury must be repaired is 0,08 %.. [26]. These ratios are lower than expected as most of the cases are not reported. Despite low prevalence, hemorrhagic-related mortality rates vary between 8% and 17% [27]. Inexperience, oversight during trocar entry, incorrect cleavage during balloon dissection and the lack of a full command of anatomy are the major causes of injury. Risk has also increased in patients who underwent abdominal surgery. All vascular structures in the groin, except the external iliac vessels, can be ligated, clipped safely or hemostasis can be achieved through the method of electrocautery sealing. Externail iliac vessel injuries require urgent repair and laparotomy should be started immediately.

b. Bladder injury:

Bladder injury is the most common complication of the urinary system. It especially occurs in the suprapubic area during trocar entry or dissection. In the event that it has been noticed during surgery, the surgeon may repair the injury laparoscopically according to his/her experience. Urinary catheters are used for 7-10 days. In the late period, patient may present with hematuria and lower abdominal pain. In these cases, the diagnosis is confirmed by a retrograde cystogram. Small defects can be treated without the need for repair through drainage of urine.

c. Bowel injury:

Bowel injuries can complicate the laparoscopic procedure. These are usually related to a dissection of the small intestine or colon attaced to the hernia sac. The sigmoid colon on the left side and the small intestine on the right side are more frequently injured. The incidence rate is about 0.13% [28]. To prevent these injuries, the digestive tract structures should be reintroduced with the peritoneum without dissecting the adhesions between the sac and the organs. Although they can occur more frequently with the TAPP technique they have also been reported for the TEP technique [29]. Other bowel injury mechanisms include direct trocar or Veress needle perforations and secondary necrosis caused by electrocoagulation. The injury can be repaired with suturing or stapling during laparoscopy. Patients with delayed bowel injury may present with peritonitis signs or sepsis one week after surgery. The mortality rate is about 4% [28].

d. Intestinal obstruction:

It is a rare complication that can occur as a result of a fascial defect larger than 5 mm which are not closed especially in the TAP procedure. Fascial defects can be easily closed with a number of devices developed by commercial medical companies. When the peritoneal layer sutured over the mesh is not fully closed it causes the migration of the intestinal tract to the preperitoneal area and therefore obstruction is unavoidable. This complication that is musc less frequent with TEP technique may develop due to an overlooked peritoneal defect.

2. Hernioplasty related complications

a. Groin pain:

Each patient's pain threshold level varies, subjective evaluation is in the forefront. If the evaluation of pain is required in terms of the success of an operation, we should be aware of the fact that chronic pain is more important than the pain in the early period. Nerve damage occurs between 2-4% and the femoral branch of genitofemoral nerve and lateral femoral cutaneal nerve are most frequently damaged [30,31]. In the literature, occurance rate of groin pain after inguinal hernia surgeries is around 11%. [32]. This problem appears as the most frequent morbidity of hernia surgery. However in the literature, in many studies groin pain is shown to be less in laparoscopic techniques. And even in a study comparing TEP procedure with Lichtenstein technique, TEP procedure is shown to be significantly superior statistically in each of the physical function, physical role, body pain, general health, and spiritual role categories [33]. Also fibrin sealant products for fixation mesh instead of the staples may decrease the groin pain.

b. Recurrence

In many studies including advanced laparoscopic centers recurrence rates were reported between 0% and 13%. It will be possible to achieve equal proportions of recurrence following impermeable open hernia repairs (tension free hernioplasty) and to obtain even lower recurrence rates with the increase of surgeons' experience and the development of laparoscopic skills. Sometimes it is not clinically evident whether swellings occured after repair are really reccurrent, a cord lipoma, a seroma or a swelling of the internal oblique muscle. In those cases extra imaging technique may be required. It is important to fully demonstrate the diagnosis of recurrence in order to avoid a second surgery in patients readmitted with inguinal pain. After the diagnosis of recurrence, most surgeons prefer open surgical method for recurrence. Nowadays, it is still controversial to consider a repeat endoscopic surgery in recurrences due to TEP or TAPP procedure.

c. Infertility

During hernia repairs, infertility problems may occur as a result of vas deferens or testicles injuries due to a traction or during dissection. Vas deferens defect may also occur during mesh fixaton. Excessive traction or long retention of vas deferens reduce the quality of sperm by disrupting the movement of sperm. Excessive fibrosis that can occur around cord depending on the type of mesh used during the repair predispose to infertility. Incidence of ductus deferens injury is 0.3% in inguinal hernia repair. [34]. To avoid this complication during hernia sac dissection, grasping the ductus deferens and excessive traction should be avoided as much as possible. Care must be taken to the surrounding structures during the placement of the mesh.

d. Orchitis

Ischemia resulting from the deterioration of testicular blood flow may cause to orchitis and then testicular atrophy. Clinical presentation is enlarged painful testicle presenting with mild fever. scrotal hematoma, seroma, hydrocele, and testicular torsion are considered at the differential diagnosis.Doppler ultrasound scan is helpful in the differential diagnosis. The way to avoid this complication is to avoid full dissection of hernia sacs with very large scrotal component. In this type of patients, hernia sac is divided just in the distal aspect of the internal ring, proximal portion is ligated with the help of Endoloop while the distal is left open. Contrary to the opinion of most surgeons, leaving the distal hernia sac open in the scrotum does not lead to an excessive increase in the formation of non-communicating hydrocele. [35]

e. The other complications:

Complications such as wound infection, seroma formation, hydrocele, development of hematoma and testicular ptosis due to the freed cremasteric muscles can be seen after endoscopic hernia repair.

f. Mesh contraction:

Mesh contraction that is shown to be responsible for some recurrence cases appears in rates up to 20%. [36]

Related with	Related with Patient	Related with	Related with mesh
Laparoscopy		hernioplasty	
Vascular injury	Ileus	Recurrence	Folding
Bowel injury	Urinary retention	Port site problems	Pai
Bladder injury	DVT	Seroma	Contraction
Gas Embolism	Cardiopulmonary complications	Hematoma	Erosion
Bowel obstruction		Hydrocele	Infection
Shoulder pain		Orchitis	Rejection
Subcutaneous emphysema		Infertility	
Arrythmias		Groin pain	
		Anesthesia, pareasthesia	
		Dysejaculation	

DVT, deep venos thrombosis

Table 1. Complications of TAPP/ TEP procedure

9. Comparison of TAPP and TEP techniques; which method is the best

When compared to TAPP procedure, advantages of TEP technique such as absence of abdominal approach, lack of risk of damage in intraperitoneal organs and vascular structures, very little risk of incisional hernia development in the port sites, absence of postoperative adhesion formation immediately come to mind. Most importantly, absence of operations such as re-suturing of the peritoneum opened during TAPP procedure may be considered as an advantage of TEP procedure. In this way, the surgery time is shortened. The main disadvantage of TEP repair is the anatomy of Retzius' space appearing complicated, a learning curve that lasts longer and relatively limited study area. Still, TEP is also contraindicated in patients with a history of prior lower abdominal surgery. However anatomy is more comprehensible and surgical area is larger in TAPP surgery. In endoscopic hernia repair, clear understanding of the anatomy of the posterior muscle is very important. TAPP technique provides greater understanding of the anatomy, as well as encourages the surgeon as initial cases. Despite all these advantages and disadvantages, in many studies comparing TEP and TAPP, obvious superiority of the two techniques to each other have not been demonstrated. [37,38]. What is

http://dx.doi.org/10.5772/57250

accepted throughout the surgical arena is that; the surgeon gets the best results in the technique that he/she develops him/herself best. We must not forget that all the surgeons involved in this domain have to knowboth techniques very well.

10. Conclusion

Although the literature on laparoscopic hernia repair is wide, except selected eligible patients, the benefit of laparoscopic procedures has not yet clearly understood, or generally accepted. However it is necessary to gain experience in laparoscopic techniques before hernia surgery. Studies showed that surgeons need to realize 30-100 operations in order to avoid recurrence and complications. [39] Laparoscopic or endoscopic groin hernia surgery is associated with short-term benefits, in terms of the postoperative pain and more rapid return to normal activities and has the advantage that it is minimal invasive compared to open mesh hernia repair but is usually performed under general anaesthesia.Unlike most surgical procedures, endoscopic groin hernioplasty has been tested in a large number of randomised controlled trials. These provide a reliable evidence base which demonstrates the feasibility and value of trials for assessing the effectiveness of laparoscopic/endoscopic procedures. For the patient to benefit from advantages of minimally invasive surgery, surgeon should either have a good knowledge on laparoscopic procecedure or transfer the patient to centers of reference in this regard. Most precisely surgeon must apply the surgical procedure he/she knows the best.

Author details

Süleyman Çetinkünar[1], Hasan Erdem[1], B. Çağlar Bilgin[2], Seyfi Emir[3], İlhan Bali[3] and Selim Sözen[3]

1 Adana Numune Training and Research Hospital, Department of General Surgery, Adana, Turkey

2 Medical Faculty of Kafkas University, Department of General Surgery, Kars, Turkey

3 Medical Faculty of Namık Kemal University, Department of General Surgery, Tekirdağ, Turkey

References

[1] Rives J, Nicaise H. A propos des hernies de l'aine et de leurs récidives. Semin Hop. 1966;31:1932-1934

[2] Stoppa R, Rives JL, Walamount C, Palot JP, Verhaege PJ, Delattre JF.The use of Dacron in the repair of hernias of the groin. Surg Clin North Am. 1984;64(2):269-285.).

[3] Bassini E. Nuovo metodo sulla cura radicale dell' ernia inguinale. Arch Soc Ital Chir. 1887:4:80

[4] Ger R, Monroe K, Duviviver R et all: Management of indirect hernias by laparoscopic closure of the neck of the sac. Am J Surg 159;370,1990

[5] Lichtenstein IL, Shulman AG, Amid PK et al. The tension free hernioplasty. Am J Surg 1989; 157:188-92

[6] Glassow WF: A comparison of the Shouldice and cooper ligament repair for adult inguinal hernias. The American Jurnal of Surgery 1976; 131: 306-311.

[7] Skandalakis. L.J. Modern Hernia Repair. 1. publ. London. Catagologing Publ. 1992.

[8] Laparoscopic techniques versus open techniques for inguinal hernia repair. Cochrane Database Syst Rev. 2003;(1):CD001785.

[9] Wantz GE: Abdominal wall hernias, in Schwartz. Ed: Seymour I. Schwartz: Principles of Surgery 7. ed Vol. 2, Bölüm 34, McGraw Hill Co, Singapore: 1999, s. 1585-1611.

[10] Skandalakis PN, Skandalakis JE, Colborn GL, Kingsnorth AN, Weidman TA, Skandalakis LJ: Abdominal wall and hernias, in Skandalakis. Ed: John E Skandalakis: Surgical Anatomy 14. ed Vol 1, Bölüm 9, PMP Co, Athens: 2004, s. 395-491.

[11] Mirilas P, Colborn GL, McClusky DA 3rd, Skandalakis LJ, Skandalakis PN, Skandalakis JE. The history of anatomy and surgery of the preperitoneal space. Arch Surg. 2005 Jan;140(1):90-4.

[12] Devlin HB, Kingsnorth A: Essential anatomy of the abdominal wall, in Devlin. Ed: H Brendan Devlin: Management of Abdominal Hernias 2. ed Bölüm 2, Chapman and Hall Co, London: 1998, s. 15-37.

[13] Milić DJ, Pejić MA. Tension-free procedures in the surgical treatment of groin hernias. Srp Arh Celok Lek. 2003 Jan-Feb;131(1-2):82-91.

[14] Bekoev VD, Kril' VA, Troianov AA, Anisimova VN, Iashchuk IuI, Blakhov NIu. Recurrence of inguinal hernia (problems and ways of treatment. Khirurgiia (Mosk). 2003;(2):45-7;

[15] Agarwal AK, Mukherjee R. Franz kaspar hasselbach (1759-1816). Indian J Surg. 2008 Apr;70(2):96-8.

[16] Chevallier JM, Wind P, Lassau JP. Damage to the inguino-femoral nerves in the treatment of hernias. An anatomical hazard of traditional and laparoscopic techniques. Ann Chir. 1996;50(9):767-75.

[17] Moreno-Egea A, Paredes PG, Perello JM. Vascular injury by tacks during totally extraperitoneal endoscopic inguinal hernioplasty.Surg Laparosc Endosc Percutan Tech. 2010 Jun;20(3):e129-31

[18] Bendavid R. The space of Bogros and the deep inguinal venous circulation. Surg Gynecol Obstet. 1992 May;174(5):355-8

[19] Nyhus LM, Condon RE, Harkins HN. Clinical experience with preperitoneal hernia repair for all types of hernia of the groin. Am J Surg. 1960;100:234-244

[20] ffect of fibrin glues on the mechanical properties of healing wounds.Byrne DJ, Hardy J, Wood RA, McIntosh R, Cuschieri ABr J Surg. 1991 Jul; 78(7):841-3

[21] Comparing sutures and human fibrin glue for mesh fixation during open inguinal hernioplasty. Sözen S, Cetinkünar S, Emir S, Yazar FM. Ann Ital Chir. 2012 Oct 2

[22] Mesh fixation with fibrin sealant during endoscopic totally extraperitoneal inguinal hernia approach: a review of 640 repairs.Berney CR, Yeo AE. Hernia. 2013 Jan 24

[23] Memon MA, Cooper NJ, Memon B, Memon MI, Abrams KR.Meta-analysis of randomized clinical trials comparing open and laparoscopic inguinal hernia repair. Br J Surg. 2003 Dec;90(12):1479-92

[24] Bittner R, Schmedt CG, Schwarz J, Kraft K, Leibl BJ. Laparoscopic transperitoneal procedure for routine repair of groin hernia. Br J Surg. 2002 Aug;89(8):1062

[25] Tamme C, Scheidbach H, Hampe C, Schneider C, Köckerling F. Totally extraperitoneal repair of recurrent inguinal hernia. Surg Endosc. 2003 Jul;17(7):1072-6. Epub 2003 May 6.).

[26] Schäfer M, Lauper M, Krähenbühl L. A nation's experience of bleeding complications during laparoscopy. Am J Surg. 2000 Jul;180(1):73-7.

[27] Olsen DO.Laparoscopic cholecystectomy. Am J Surg. 1991 Mar;161(3):339-44.

[28] Van der Voort M, Heijnsdijk EA, Gouma DJ. Bowel injury as a complication of laparoscopy. Br J Surg. 2004 Oct;91(10):1253-8.

[29] Ramshaw BJ, Tucker JG, Conner T, Mason EM, Duncan TD, Lucas GW. A comparison of the approaches to laparoscopic herniorrhaphy. Surg Endosc 1996;10:29-32

[30] Tam KW, Liang HH, Chai CY. Outcomes of staple fixation of mesh versus nonfixation in laparoscopic total extraperitoneal inguinal repair: a meta-analysis of randomized controlled trials. World J Surg. 2010 Dec;34(12):3065-74

[31] Stark E, Oestreich K, Wendl K, Rumstadt B, Hagmüller E. Nerve irritation after laparoscopic hernia repair. Surg Endosc. 1999 Sep;13(9):878-81.

[32] Poobalan AS, Bruce J, Smith WC, King PM, Krukowski ZH, Chambers WA. A review of chronic pain after inguinal herniorrhaphy. Clin J Pain. 2003 Jan-Feb;19(1):48-54

[33] Myers E, Browne KM, Kavanagh DO, Hurley M. Laparoscopic (TEP) versus Lichtenstein inguinal hernia repair: a comparison of quality-of-life outcomes. World J Surg. 2010 Dec;34(12):3059-64

[34] Sheynkin YR, Hendin BN, Schlegel PN, Goldstein M. Microsurgical repair of iatrogenic injury to the vas deferens. J Urol. 1998 Jan;159(1):139-41

[35] Fong Y, Wantz GE. Prevention of ischemic orchitis during inguinal hernioplasty. Surg Gynecol Obstet. 1992 May;174(5):399-402.

[36] Amid PK. How to avoid recurrence in Lichtenstein tension-free hernioplasty. Am J Surg. 2002 Sep;184(3):259-60

[37] Laparoscopic surgery for inguinal hernia repair:Technology appraisal 83, London,UK, 2007, National Institute for Clinical Excellence

[38] McCormack K, Wake BL, Fraser C, Vale L, Perez J, Grant A. Transabdominal pre-peritoneal (TAPP) versus totally extraperitoneal (TEP) laparoscopic techniques for inguinal hernia repair: a systematic review. Hernia. 2005 May;9(2):109-14. Epub 2005 Feb 10.

[39] Wake BL, McCormack K, Fraser C, Vale L, Perez J, Grant A. Transabdominal pre-peritoneal (TAPP) vs totally extraperitoneal (TEP) laparoscopic techniques for inguinal hernia repair. Cochrane Database Syst Rev. 2005;25:CD004703

Chapter 3

Laparoscopic Approach in the Treatment of Inguinal Hernia and Associated Pathologies in Children

Antonio Marte, Gianpaolo Marte and
Pio Parmeggiani

Additional information is available at the end of the chapter

http://dx.doi.org/10.5772/57158

1. Introduction

Inguinal hernia is one of the most common surgical disorders in children. Galen first, in 176 A.D, described the processus vaginalis as "The duct descending to the testicle is a small offshoot of the great peritoneal sac in the lower abdomen". The surgical history of inguinal hernias dates back to ancient Egypt. From Bassini's heralding of the modern era to today's mesh-based open and laparoscopic repairs, this history closely resembles the evolution in anatomical understanding and development of the techniques of general surgery. Ferguson, in 1899, proposed hernia repair by just exposure, dissection, simple high ligation and removal of the hernia sac, and this was applied successfully to the pediatric population by Potts et al. [1-3] Fig 1-2-3

While in adult hernia repairs, the underlying principle involved reconstruction of weakened muscles and aponeurosis in multiple anatomical layers, for pediatric hernia simple dissection and high ligation of processus vaginalis at internal ring was found to be sufficient to provide a long lasting cure to repair indirect inguinal hernia. The Ferguson principle still remains the basis of all pediatric hernia repairs even in the 21st century. With advances in operating techniques, better suture materials and pediatric anesthesia, the ferguson principle remains at the basis of laparoscopic hernia repair.

The evolution reached its current level in 1990 shortly after the introduction of laparoscopic cholecystectomy, when the laparoscopic approach to inguinal hernia repair was introduced. [4]

In the last few years the use of the laparoscopic approach to inguinal hernia has increased not only for accurate diagnoses, but also for treatment.

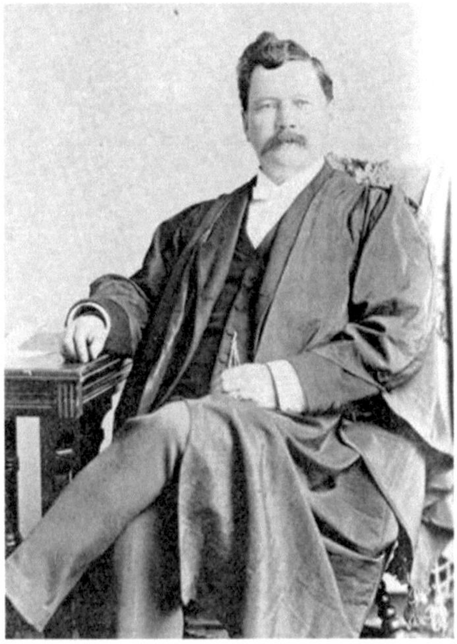

Figure 1. Alexander Hugh Ferguson (1853-1911).

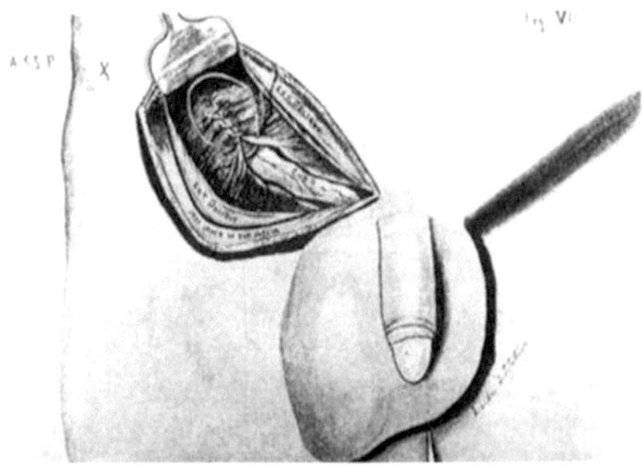

Figure 2. The original drawing of Ferguson technique.

The data reported in the literature underline the safety, reproducibility and excellent cosmetic results of this technique to an extent that it can now be considered as a valid alternative to traditional surgery and a first choice technique to explore the contralateral side, in the differential diagnosis between direct and indirect hernias, and for the treatment of recurrences [5-8]. Nevertheless some perplexity still remains about the higher percentage of recurrence rate with this technique ranging from 3.4% to 4.1% compared to the open technique. [3-6]

We present here our experience with the laparoscopic inguinal hernia repair in children with the addition of the lateral incision of the sac and the suture of the inner inguinal ring. As many

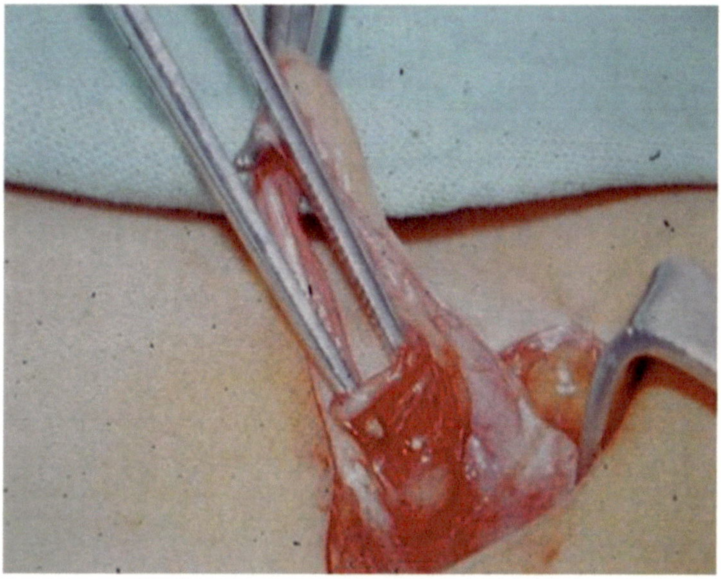

Figure 3. Traditional open inguinal herniotomy in children.

as 220 patients were operated on from January 2004 to June 2012. The age ranged from 2 months to 12 years (mean, 2.5 years), with a follow-up between 1 and 7 years (mean 3.5 yrs). There were 90 bilateral and 130 unilateral inguinal hernia, male/female ratio 141/79.

All the procedures were performed under general anaesthesia and by the same surgeon (AM). Inclusion criteria included bilateral inguinal hernia, recurrent hernia, hernia in obese children, incarcerated hernia, and ipsilateral hernia with questionable hernia on the contralateral side. Exclusion criteria included patients with undescended testicles or who have had many abdominal surgeries.

According to the age, patients were either asked to urinate before the operation or underwent manual bladder voiding after the anaesthesia. In the early experience a Veress needle was employed to induce pneumoperitoneum (12 mmHg) with carbon dioxide (CO_2); the Veress was subsequently replaced by a 5 mm reusable Hasson trocar introduced by "open technique". This resulted useful not only for safety but also in case of associated umbilical hernia or previous surgical procedure, to prevent injuring the adherent bowel or omentum. The 5mm 0° or 30° laparoscope was employed first to explore the abdominal cavity, and then to ensure patency of the processus vaginalis on both sides. Thereafter, two operating 2 mm or 3 mm reusable trocars were inserted in the lower right and left quadrants of the abdominal wall, along the midclavear line; the patient was then placed in mild Trendelenburg position. (Fig 4) The procedure usually required a needle holder, a grasper and a pair of scissors. The suture needle was introduced in the cavity through the abdominal wall, above the inguinal ring. The sac was previously incised for 1 to 2 cm laterally from the inner inguinal ring to the distal part of the sac exposing a triangular area or removing a small portion of peritoneum (IRIS Technique – Inguinal Ring Incision Suture) (fig 5), then the inner inguinal ring was closed adopting a W-shaped suture or a purse string using non absorbable, 3/0 - 4/0 polybutester monofilament on a 17/20-mm swaged needle, starting from the lateral side, grabbing some underlying tissue, to the medial one. A return stitch was then placed near the first lateral access to obtain a tension-free knot. Four to five intracorporeal knots were always placed to ensure closure. Great care was used to close the medial margin of the inguinal ring to prevent recurrence. The vas deferens and testicular vessels in male patients were completely untouched and safeguarded. If necessary a second stitch has been applied to not put stress on the previous one with excessive tension. The needle was retrieved through the working port, and the umbilical wound was then closed with absorbable sutures while the lateral wounds were just approximated. (Fig 5 to 11)

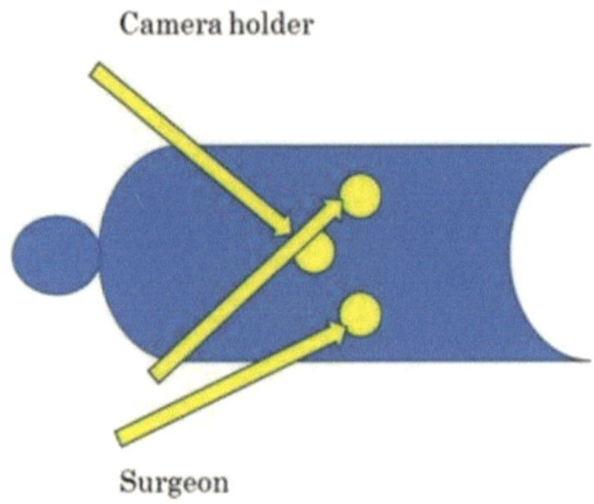

Figure 4. Theater layout, trocar placement.

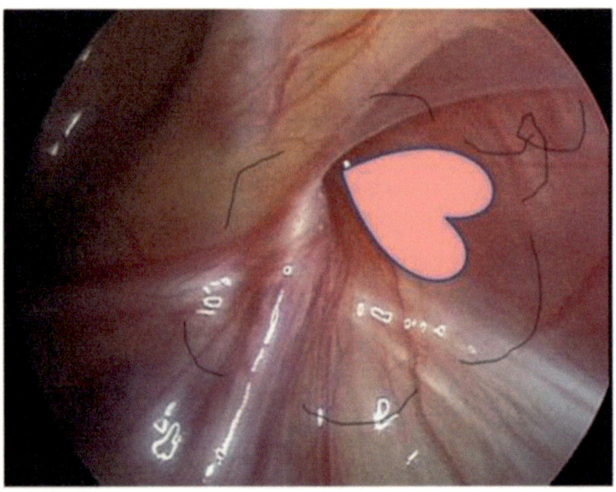

Figure 5. Scheme of the peritoneum incision/ purse-string suture.

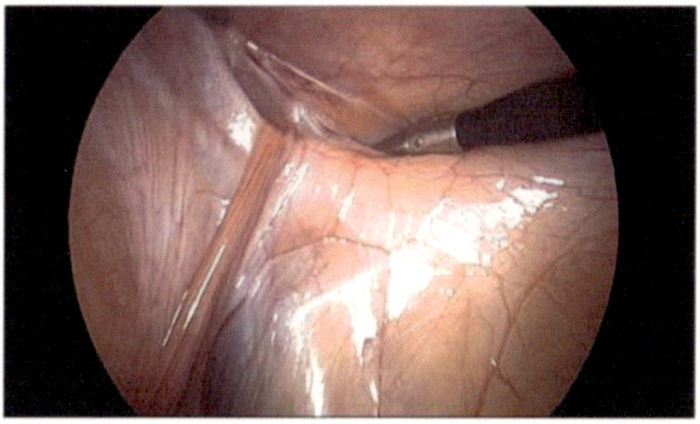

Figure 6. Laparoscopic step of the incision of the sac: Incision/removal of a small lateral portion of the sac.

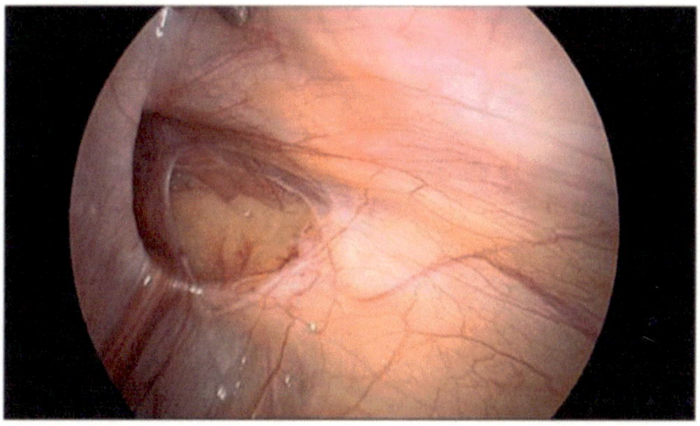

Figure 7. Triangular area peritoneum – free.

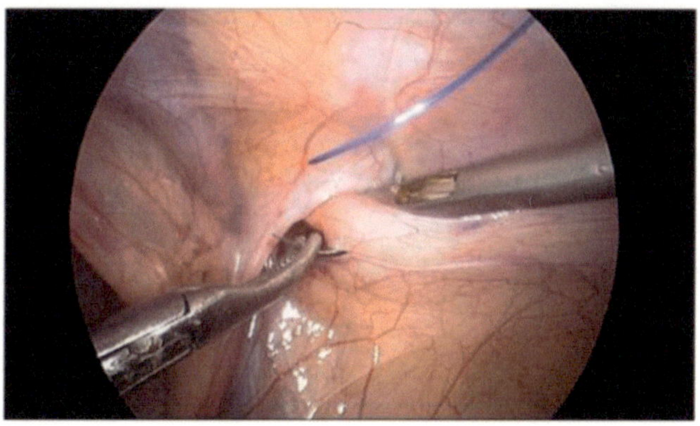

Figure 8. Starting suture from the lateral part of the sac.

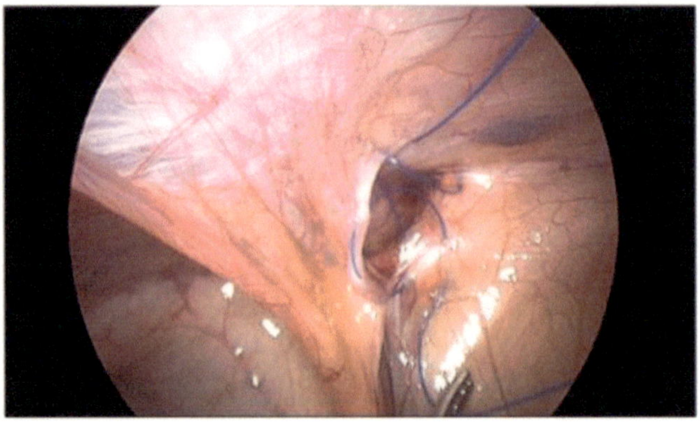

Figure 9. Completion of the purse string suture.

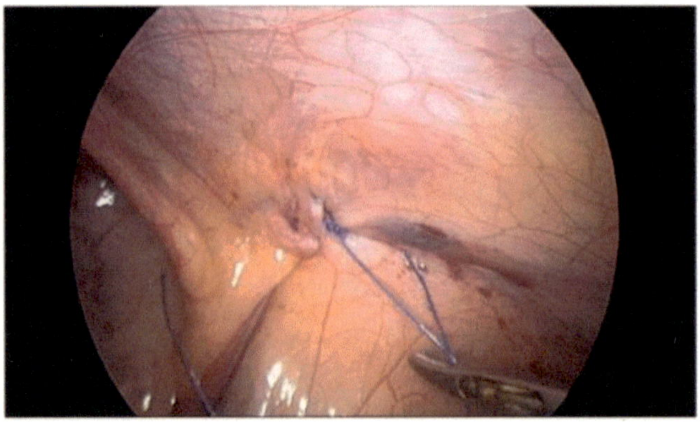

Figure 10. Final view of the closure of the inguinal ring.

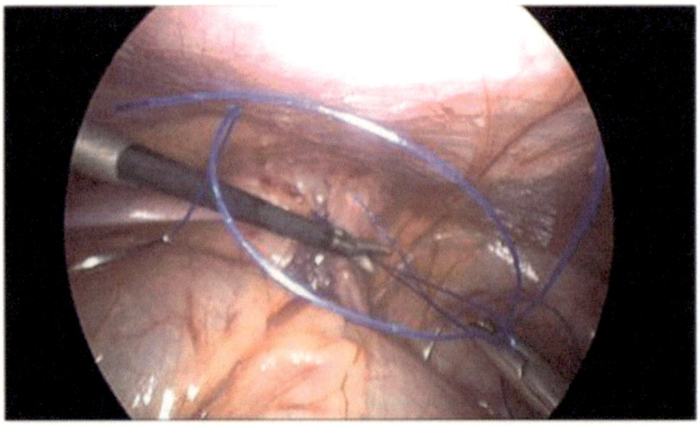

Figure 11. Herniorraphy on the contralateral side.

At the end of the procedure, the skin was closed with adhesive strips and the umbilical fascia was closed with polyglactin 3/0 suture at the end of the procedure. The associated umbilical hernias were treated in the usual way closing the fascial defect in a transverse direction with interrupted absorbable polyglactin suture. In some cases, there was need for only one administration of acetaminophen in the first few post operative hours.

Mean operative time was 19±3 m′ in the monolateral hernia group and 28±4 m′ in the bilateral hernia group. Longer time was required in cases of treatment of adhesions or associated pathologies. The majority of patients was discharged the same day or the next day scheduling the revaluation at 1 week, 6 months and 1 year. Bilateral inguinal hernia was present in 6.5%. A contralateral patent ductus was present in 17%. No patient required an additional port or conversion to open procedure. A slight bleeding occurred in some patients at insertion port side without sequelae. In the immediate postoperative time, 20 patients presented mild emphysema on a portal site or at scrotal level, which resolved spontaneously. 2 (0.9%) patients, in the present series, after the adoption of incision/suture of the internal inguinal ring, developed recurrence after a period varying between 1 and 6 weeks, which was repaired with standard open surgery in 1 case and laparoscopically in the other. No patient presented postoperative complications including testicular atrophy, wound infection or incision site herniation. No metachronous hernia occurred during the follow-up (mean follow-up: 3,5 yrs). [9] The associated diseases treated in the same session has been as follows: umbilical hernia 31 pts. ; incarcerated hernia 18 pts; hydrocele15 pts; incarcerated omentum 12 pts, varicocele 8 pts, incarcerated ovary 1 pt; intestinal adhesions1 pt. (Figs. 12 to 14) The technique has undergone the following changes: passage to the open technique for the insertion of the first trocar after a period of use of the Veress. Use of incision and removal of a wedge of the parietal peritoneum at the level of the inner inguinal ring to promote healing. Use of a W-shaped or purse string suture to tie on the same side. Reinforcement, when necessary, of the suture with the overlapping of lateral ligaments. Simple interrupted stitches have been used only to reinforce the running or purse string suture.

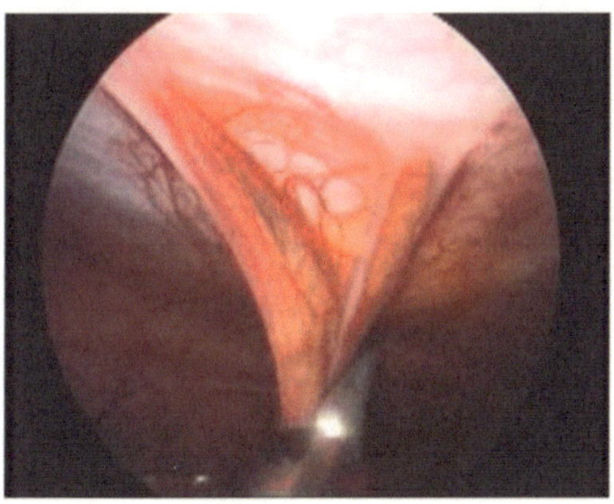

Figure 12. Adhesiolysis during laparoscopic herniorraphy

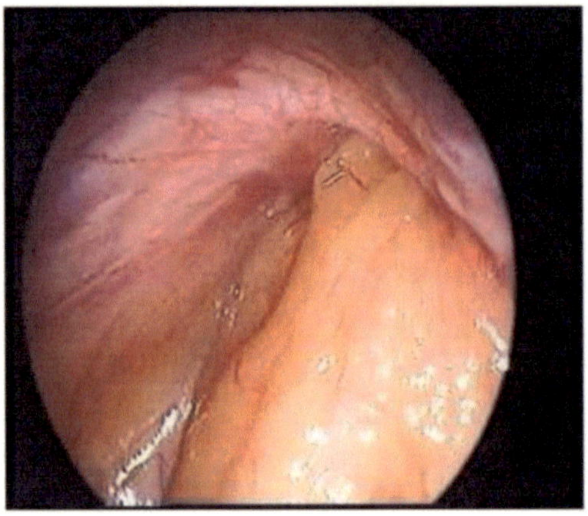

Figure 13. Laparoscopic view of the incarcerated omentum

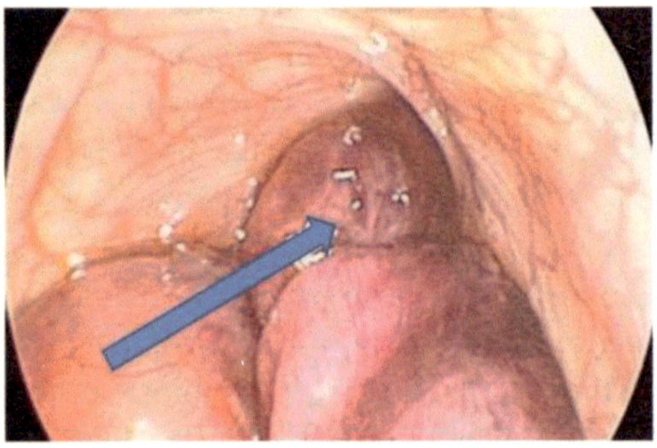

Figure 14. Laparoscopic view of an incarcerated hernia

2. Discussion

In our experience the results of laparoscopic approach to inguinal hernia and some associated pathologies in children with IRIS technique are safe, easy and versatile and the section of the outer portion of the internal inguinal ring looks like a useful device in reducing relapses.

Different techniques has been described for tightening up the hernia opening by laparoscopy with varied results. [10] They include the following techniques:

1. Intracorporeal suturing and knotting technique

This has been the initial method adopted at the inception of laparoscopic inguinal hernia repair in children thanks to the reports by Schier an Montupet. The technique employs three ports and uses nonabsorbable suture materials. In this method, intraperitoneal suture of the internal inguinal ring is performed to close the processus vaginalis at its origin. The closure is achieved by suturing in N, W or purse-string fashion and knotting tight the internal inguinal ring with 1 or 2 stitches. Sometimes simple interrupted stitches can be utilized to close the ring. This method has a certain recurrence rate (0–5.7%) and good intracorporeal laparoscopic knotting skill is required.

More recently, with refinements in technology, the single procedure is currently attracting attention. In their experience with modified single-port laparoscopic procedures in children, Rothenberg *et al*. found very encouraging outcome. This report corroborates with a study by Chang on technical refinements in single-port laparoscopic surgery of inguinal hernia in infants and children. In a comparison study by Bharathi *et al.*, single-port technique was preferred to the three port due to better outcome. Of course this technique presents technical difficulties compared to the classic three-port procedure. [11-13]

2. Inversion and ligation technique

This method of laparoscopic inguinal repair is widely used in girls. This is a modification of the intracorporeal technique, using three ports and nonabsorbable sutures. It is thought that inversion and ligation of sac at the internal inguinal ring would reduce the risk of recurrence (0.8–2.5%).The problems faced in the intracorporeal technique may also apply here. In 2009, some Authors described the selective sac extraction method for inguinal hernia repair in children by minimally invasive procedure with satisfactory surgical and cosmetic outcome. In the sac extraction technique, the sac is extracted and ligated openly. In the inversion and ligation technique, the sac is isolated, inverted, and ligated laparoscopically. [14-17]

3. Complete resection with or without ligation technique

This is an emerging technique and represents another modification of the intracorporeal technique, with three ports and nonabsorbable sutures employed. In this technique, the hernia sac is resected and closed with a purse-string suture at the level of the internal inguinal ring. The efficacy of this technique is attributed to the fact that in this procedure, the sac is wholly resected and this section favors the healing without leaving skip portions as happens in the intracorporeal suture. The skip portions, especially at the medial aspect of internal inguinal ring, should account for some of the recurrences in some reports. [18]

With resection and no ligation technique the hernia sac is resected at the level of the internal inguinal and allowed to close spontaneously. This technique has been reported in literature with preliminary results showing satisfactory outcome and no recurrence. The method uses three ports and no sutures are employed.[19]

4. Flip-flap technique

In this procedure, a flip-flap is raised in the internal inguinal ring and used to close the defect. The hernia opening is repaired with a peritoneal flip-flap anchored with a single tension-free intracorporeal suture. The vas and testicular vessel remain completely untouched. The valve mechanism, according to these Authors, avoid scrotal collection and prevent hernia recurrence. This is a three-port technique that uses absorbable sutures. Yip *et al*. did not record any recurrence with this technique. Satisfactory results have been noticed by Hassan *et al.* in a comparative study of this flip-flap technique with the conventional open technique. [20,21]

5. Extracorporeal suturing

This method is currently being adopted by increasing number of pediatric surgeons particularly because has low recurrence rates (0–2.0%), and more importantly, knotting does not require any special skill because it is done externally in the subcutaneous tissue in the conventional manner. The low recurrence rate in this technique is attributed to the fact that in this procedure the sac is wholly ligated without leaving skip portions. The limitation of this technique is that special needles and introducers are required. In the review, spinal needle, special 19-gauge needle, hook, and host of other instruments are currently being used with good outcome. [22,23,24]

6. Use of tissue adhesives

A useful device to reinforce the suture the internal inguinal ring can be represented by the application of tissue glue.

Initial animal experimental studies showed that tissue adhesives could be used in tissue approximation. Further, experimental animal models have continued to establish the role of tissue adhesives in inguinal hernia repair. Today tissue adhesive is being employed in a lot of laparoscopic procedures including inguinal hernia repair [25-29].

All these artifices indicate that the LH is a technique still in evolution and the near zero recurrence, if possible, is a goal not completely achieved. In our previous experience the sole W-shaped suture was associated to a 3.75% of recurrences [30-32]. The lateral incision with blunt dissection of peritoneum before suturing the inguinal ring resulted, instead, in a significant improvement of the outcome. These results, which are in line with those obtained by other Authors, could be due to a better sealing of the internal inguinal ring obtained after the incision of the peritoneum. [33] We think in fact that, at present, the real problem that all these technical changes would assume that partial or total peritoneum incision practiced at the level of internal inguinal ring can foster internal inguinal ring closure itself. But although the results are better and the comparison result favorable to this techniques there is not a clear demonstration of why and whether, on the long term, relapses are really reduced. In any case laparoscopic optic magnification allows to surgeon to dissect and handle the vas and the vessels very easily. In the open technique, the vas deferens is very vulnerable to mechanical injury, and the incidence of vas injury may be underestimated because the incidence of unilateral vas deferens obstruction was reported to be 26.7% for a subfertile patient with a history of open inguinal hernia surgery in childhood [34-36].

Moreover the possibility of recognize a contralateral patent processus vaginalis can play a role in preventing metachronous hernias. This does not mean that this condition represents a future inguinal hernia but since the adoption of this procedure the number of metachronous hernias was reduced. [37]

3. Conclusion

The data from our follow-up confirm that the results of the laparoscopic IRIS technique, presents an acceptable low percentage of recurrences that is comparable to those of the open technique, with the advantage of reduced post operative pain, rapid return to everyday activities, and optimal cosmetic results. Although the results of our experience seems promising we think that the follow-up is too short and the number of the patients too small for drawing definitive conclusion.

Author details

Antonio Marte, Gianpaolo Marte and Pio Parmeggiani

*Address all correspondence to: antonio.marte@unina2.it

Second University of Naples, Pediatric Surgery, Naples, Italy

References

[1] Vessella A, Marte A, Parmeggiani P. (2005) Terapia dell'ernia inguinale nel bambino. Dal Papiro di Ebers alla Laparoscopia. Una storia affascinante. p. 1-87. Laruffa Editore,Reggio Calabria. ISBN: 88-7221-281-2

[2] Ferguson AH. Oblique inguinal hernia: A typical operation for its radical cure. JAMA 1899; 33:6-14.

[3] Potts WJ, Riker WL, Lewis JE. The treatment of inguinal hernia in infants and children. Ann Surg 1950; 132:566-576

[4] Schier F. Laparoscopic herniorrhaphy in girls. J Pediatr Surg. 1998;33(10):1495–1497.

[5] Mintelburg D.M., Nuchtern j.G., Jaksic t. et al: Laparoscopic evaluation of the pediatric inguinal hernia – a meta-analysis. J Pediatr Surg 1998, 33: 874 -8.

[6] Saranga Bharathi R, Arora M, Baskaran V.Pediatric Inguinal Hernia: Laparoscopic Versus Open Surgery JSLS. 2008 Jul-Sep; 12(3): 277–281.

[7] Gorsler C.M., Schier F.: Laparoscopic herniorraphy in children. Surg. Endosc 2003 17:571 -

[8] Schier F. Laparoscopic inguinal hernia repair – a prospective personal series of 542 children. J Pediatr surg 2006;41: 1081-4

[9] Schier F, Montoupet P, Esposito C. Laparoscopic Inguinal Herniorraphy in Children: A Three Center Experience With 933 Repairs. J Pediatr Surg 2002; 37: 395-7

[10] Marte A, Sabatino MD, Borrelli M, Parmeggiani P. Decreased recurrence rate in the laparoscopic herniorraphy in children: comparison between two techniques. J Laparoendosc Adv Surg Tech A. 2009 Apr;19(2):259-62. doi: 10.1089/lap.2008.0292

[11] Christopher S. Lukong CS.Surgical Techniques of Laparoscopic Inguinal Hernia Repair in Childhood: A Critical Appraisal J Surg Tech Case Rep. 2012 Jan-Jun; 4(1): 1–5. doi: 10.4103/2006-8808.100343

[12] Rothenberg SS, Shipman K, Yoder S. Experience with modified single port laparoscopic procedures in children. J Laparoendosc Adv Surg Tech. 2009;19:695–8. 11. Chang YT. Technical refinements in single port laparoscopic surgery of inguinal hernia in infants and children. DiagTherEndosc. 2010;2010:392847.

[13] Bharathi RS, Dabas AK, Arora M, Baskaran V. Laparoscopic ligationof internal ring-three port versus single port technique. Are working ports necessary? J LaparoendoscAdvSurg Tech A. 2008;18:891–4.

[14] Lipskar AM, Soffer SZ, Glick RD, Rosen NG, Levitt MA, Hong AR. Laparoscopic inguinal hernia inversion and ligation in female children: A review of 173 consecutive cases at a single institution. JPediatrSurg. 2010;45:1370–4.

[15] Guner YS, Emami CN, Chokshi NK, Wang K, Shin CE. Inversion herniotomy: A laparoscopic technique for female inguinal hernia repair. J Laparoendosc Adv Surg Tech. 2010;20:481–4.

[16] Zallen G, Glick PL. Laparoscopic inversion and ligation inguinal hernia repair in girls. J LaparoendoscAdvSurg Tech A. 2007;17:143–5.

[17] Ikeda H, Hatanaka M, Suzuki M, Fuji J, Takara K, Ishimara Y. Selective sac extraction method: Another minimally invasive procedure for inguinal hernia repair in children: A technical innovation with satisfactory surgical and cosmetic outcome. J Pediatr Surg. 2009;44:1666–71.

[18] Riquelme M, Aranda A, Riquelme QM. Laparoscopic pediatric inguinal hernia repair: No ligation, just resection. J LaparoendoscAdvSurg Tech A. 2010;20:77–80.

[19] Yip KF, Tam PK, Li MK. Laparoscopic flip-flap hernioplasty: An innovative technique for pediatric hernia surgery. SurgEndosc. 2004;18:1126–9.

[20] Hassan ME, Mustafawi AR. Laparoscopic flip-flap technique versus conventional inguinal hernia repair in children. JSLS. 2007;11:90–3.

[21] Kellnar S. Percutaneous laparoscopic hernia repair in children. Zentralbl.Chir. 2009;134:542–4.

[22] Dutta S, Albanese C. Transcutaneous laparoscopic hernia repair in children: A prospective review of 275 hernia repair with minimium 2 year follow up. Surg Endosc. 2009; 23:103–7.

[23] Uchida H, Kawashima H, Goto C, Sato K, Yoshida M, Takazawa S, et al. Inguinal hernia repair in children using single-incision laparoscopic-assisted percutaneous extraperitoneal closure. J Pediatr Surg. 2010;45:2386–9.

[24] Harrison MR, Lee H, Albanese CT, Farmer DL. Subcutaneous endoscopically assisted ligation (SEAL) of the internal ring for repair of inguinal hernias in children: a novel technique. J Pediatr Surg. 2005 Jul;40(7):1177-80.

[25] Olguner M, Aktuq T, Akqur FM, Pabuccuoglu U. Experimental study investigating the feasibility of new method for laparoscopic indirect hernia repair. J InvestSurg. 1997;10:189–92.

[26] Kato Y, Yamataka A, Miyano G, Tei E, Koga H, Lane GJ, et al. Tissue adhesives for repairing inguinal hernia: A preliminary study. J Laparoendosc Adv Surg Tech. 2005;15:424–8

[27] Turial S, Kreutz M, Hausser S, Enders J, Schier F. CD rats as an animal model in the experimental study of laparoscopic hernia repair. Eur J PediatrSurg. 2010;20:330–3.

[28] Cushieri A. Tissue adhesives in endosurgery. Semin Laparosc Surg. 2001;8:63–8.

[29] Esposito C, Damiano K, Settimi A, De Marco M, Maglio P, Centonze A. Experience with use of tissue adhesives in pediatric endoscopic surgery. SurgEndosc. 2004;18:290–2.

[30] Chan K.L., Tam P.K.H.: Technical refinements in laparoscopic repair of childhood inguinal hernias. Surg Endosc 2004 18: 957 – 60.

[31] Chan KL, Chan HY, Hang Tam PK. Towards a near –zero recurrence rate in laparoscopic inguinal hernia repair for pediatric patients of all age. J Pediatr Surg 2007 42, 1993 – 1997

[32] Schier F. Laparoscopic repair of inguinal hernias in Atlas of Pediatric laparoscopy and thoracoscopy. Edited by G.W. Holcomb III, K. E. Georgeson, S. S. Rothenberg. Saunders Elsevier. 2008. Pag: 195-198

[33] Montupet P, Esposito C.Fifteen years experience in laparoscopic inguinal hernia repair in pediatric patients. Results and considerations on a debated procedure. Surg Endosc. 2011 Feb;25(2):450-3. doi: 10.1007/s00464-010-1188-6. Epub 2010 Jun 2

[34] Matsuda T. Diagnosis and treatment of post-herniorrhaphy vas deferens obstruction. Int J Urol 2000 May; 7 Suppl: S35-8

[35] Matsuda T, Muguruma K, Hiura Y, Okuno H, Shichiri Y, Yoshida O. Seminal tract obstruction caused by childhood inguinal herniorrhaphy: results of microsurgical reanastomosis. J Urol. 1998 Mar;159(3):837-40

[36] Matsuda T, Horii Y, Yoshida O. Unilateral obstruction of the vas deferens caused by childhood inguinal herniorraphy in male infertility patients. Fertil Steril 1992; 58: 609-613

[37] Choi W, Hall NJ, Garriboli M, Ron O, Curry JI, Cross K, Drake DP, Kiely EM, Eaton S, De Coppi P, Pierro A. Outcomes following laparoscopic inguinal hernia repair in infants compared with older children. Pediatr Surg Int. 2012 Dec;28(12):1165-9.

Chapter 4

Laparoscopic Approach to Incarcerated/Sliding Indirect Inguinal Hernia in Children in Comparison with Open Approach

Masao Endo, Michinobu Ohno, Fumiko Yoshida, Miwako Nakano, Toshihiko Watanabe and Etsuji Ukiyama

Additional information is available at the end of the chapter

http://dx.doi.org/10.5772/58285

1. Introduction

Usual elective open herniorrhaphy for pediatric indirect inguinal hernia is technically easy, with little variation. It becomes, however, much more difficult and troublesome, with a high incidence of postoperative complications, when the hernia contains incarcerated and/or sliding viscera [1 – 3].

Although the laparoscopic approach during pediatric herniorrhaphy has flourished world-wide, analysis of cohorts of hernia patients with incarcerated/sliding viscera or comparisons between traditional open herniorrhaphy and the laparoscopic approach have been scarce. The laparoscopic approach to such conditions is considered theoretically superior in terms of identifying the correct relation of the anatomic structures under direct vision [4 – 6]. The purpose of this paper is to analyze findings on indirect hernias with incarceration/sliding and to validate the efficacy of the laparoscopic approach in comparison with the open approach.

2. Materials and method

A consecutive series of 91 children with incarcerated/sliding hernia (I/SH), chosen from among 1, 768 children with indirect inguinal hernia/hydrocele, experienced during 11 years, were analyzed. The cohort consisted of 1, 043 boys and 725 girls, 83 with bilateral hernia, 1, 023 with right hernia and 662 with left. Open herniorrhaphy (OH) with/without diagnostic laparoscopy or laparoscopic herniorrhaphy (LH) was selected according to parental preference under informed consent. Medical records of children with I/SH were selected and analyzed in terms of distribution of sex, age, kinds of viscera contained in the sac, operation time, intraoperative findings, and complications between OH and LH groups. Data from the whole cohort (WC) served as control. Children whose I/SH were solved by manual reduction before the operation were excluded from the analysis. Twenty patients who had complex procedures during the period of development of LH were excluded from the analysis and patients who underwent combined procedures affecting definitive herniorrhaphy were also excluded from the analysis of the operation time.

[Statistical analysis] Continuous data were expressed as the mean+/ – standard deviation (SD). Statistical significance was calculated using a two – tailed *t* – test. For proportional data, the chi – square test was used.

Operation method: In LH, bilateral internal inguinal rings (IIRs) and the condition of prolapsed viscera were inspected using a 5 mm laparoscope inserted through an umbilical incision with the assistance of a 2 mm grasper inserted through a stab wound in the midline just below the umbilicus. After the hernial content was reduced by a combined technique of external manual pressure and internal lead with a grasper, a circuit suture was placed around the IIR using an Endoneedle technique and knotted extracorporeally, resulting in complete closure of the IIR without any skip area. In female patients, after reducing the prolapsed viscera back into the peritoneal cavity, a circuit suture was placed distal to the U – turned Fallopian tube. The details of the patent processus vaginalis (PPV) closure have been described in a previous report [7, 8]. For infants below the age of 1y 6m, the IIR was closed with double ligation [7]. If a contra – lateral PPV (cPPV) was identified, it was closed.

In OH, the traditional procedure described in reference [9] was performed through a crease incision on the affected side. The hernial sac was opened and the prolapsed organ was pushed back into the abdomen. When a cPPV was noted by diagnostic laparoscopy via ipsilateral hernia sac, it was closed through a crease incision. For ovary/adnexa – containing inguinal hernia, IIR was closed using a modified Woolley technique [10] (Fig. 1).

3. Results

Demographic data of the patients are listed in Table 1. Ages in I/SH group averaged 1y11m in contrast to 3y10m in the WC ($p<0.05$). There were six patients with sliding or incarcerated cecum/appendix (0.3% of WC), 14 with incarcerated bowel loops (0.8%), 18 with incarcerated omentum (1.0%) and 53 with sliding/incarcerated ovary/adnexa (3.0% of WC and 7.3% of total girls). The average ages of the cecum/appendix group, the bowel loops group and the ovary/adnexa group were 8, 9 and 7 months, respectively. The ages of children with omental incarceration were different from those with other visceral incarceration/sliding (6y10m on average; $p<0.01$). Distinct distribution by sex was characteristic among kinds of contained viscera. Thirty – two I/SH (35.6%) were found in boys and 59 (64.8%) in girls. Of 725 hernias

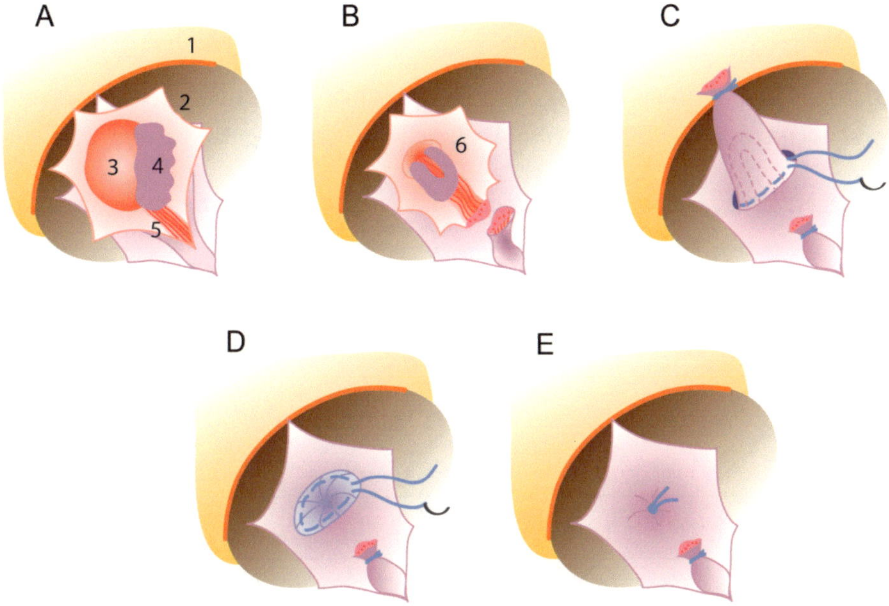

Figure 1. Modified Wooley technique. Incarcerated ovary and fimbria are seen in the opened hernial sac (A). The ovary and fimbria have been pushed back into the peritoneal space. U – turned Fallopian tube remains in the sac. The round ligament is divided (B). The hernial sac is closed and ligated distal to the U – turned Fallopian tube. A purse – string suture is placed around the neck of the hernial sac (C). The proximal sac is then invaginated into the peritoneal cavity through the internal ring (D). The Purse – string suture is ligated. Z – suture placed through the transversals fascia is added if needed for tight closure. Numbers indicate; 1, upper leaf of the incision; 2, opened hernial sac; 3, ovary; 4, fimbria; 5, round ligament; 6, Fallopian tube.

in girls, 59 (8.1%) presented with I/SH, whereas, of 1, 043 hernias in boys, 32 (0.1%) presented with I/SH, suggesting a higher incidence of I/SH in girls than in boys ($p<0.05$). There was male preponderance accounting for 84.2% of group cecum/appendix, omentum and bowel loops. Laterality of hernia appearance showed right – side preponderance in the WC (bilateral 4.7%, right 57.9%, left 37.4%), while the I/SH group showed various distributions. Cecum/appendix incarceration/sliding was seen in the right – side group only; omental incarceration was seen in the right – and left – side groups at nearly equal rates, while bowel loops and ovary/adnexa revealed left – side preponderance (64% and 55%, respectively).

Distribution of operative procedures is seen in Table 2. Among 91 patients with S/IH, 76 (5.3% of whole LH) underwent LH and 15 (4.8% of whole OH) underwent OH (statistically not significant). LH/OH ratio in S/IH was compatible with those in the WC. The OH group consisted of one patient in each group, cecum/appendix, bowel loops and omentum, respectively. In the ovary/adnexa group, the LH/OH ratio (LH:OH=1:0.3) was compatible with those in the WC (1:0.2).

Mean operation time in the OH group was longer than in the LH group (53.7 minutes vs. 38.0). The difference between the LH and OH groups was statistically significant ($p<0.01$). Furthermore, the operation time in the OH group exceeded the averaged operation time of bilateral

OH in the WC (47.4 minutes, p<0.05), while in the LH group it was 38.0 minutes, resembling the bilateral LH in the WC (37.6 minutes) (Table 3). Regarding intraoperative complication, one girl in the OH group had an injury to the Fallopian tube and underwent anastomosis under a surgical microscope. Other major complications were not recognized in either group.

	Number	Age (year)	Sex	Sites
	(ratio to WC, %)	(mean +/ – SD)	male : female	right : left : bilateral
Whole cohort (WC)	1,768	3.8 +/ – 3.0	1.0 : 0.7	1.0 : 0.7 : 0.1
Incarceration/sliding	91 (5.1)	1.9 +/ – 2.9	1.0 : 1.8	1.0 : 1.0 : 0.1
Cecum/appendix	6 (0.3)	0.7 +/ – 0.6	1.0 : 0.00	1.0 : 0.0 : 0.0
Bowel loops	14 (0.8)	0.8 +/ – 0.8	1.0 : 0.08	1.0 : 1.8 : 0.3
Omentum	18 (1.0)	6.8 +/ – 2.8	1.0 : 0.04	1.0 : 0.9 : 0.1
Ovary/adnexa	53 (3.0, 7.3*)	0.6 +/ – 0.8	0.0 : 1.00	1.0 : 1.2 : 0.1

Note: *, ratio to total numbers of girl in the WC

Table 1. Demographic data of patients.

	Operative procedure				
	LH	LH : OH	OH	miscellaneous	Total
Whole cohort (WC)	1,438	1.0 : 0.2	310	20	1,768
Incarceration/sliding	76	1.0 : 0.2	15	0	91
Cecum/appendix	5	1.0 : 0.2	1		6
Bowel loops	13	1.0 : 0.08	1		14
Omentum	17	1.0 : 0.06	1		18
Ovary/adnexa	41	1.0 : 0.3	12		53

Abbreviations: LH, laparoscopic herniorrhaphy; OH, open herniorrhaphy

Table 2. Distribution of operative procedures.

	LH		OH
	(minutes, mean +/ – SD)		(minutes, mean +/ – SD)
Whole cohort *	37.6 +/ – 13.9 (n=623)	P<0.01**	47.4 +/ – 19.8 (n=62)
	n.s.***		p<0.05***
Incarceration/sliding	38.0 +/ – 11.8 (n=73)	P<0.01**	53.7 +/ – 22.7 (n=12)

Note: *, operation time for bilateral repair; **, statistical difference between LH and OH;

***, statistical difference between whole cohort and Incarceration/sliding; n.s., not significant

Table 3. Operation times.

http://dx.doi.org/10.5772/58285

4. Characteristic findings according to the prolapsing viscera.

4.1. Cecum/appendix

Five of six patients underwent LH. Three exhibited appendicial sliding only. One of two boys with LH had a mesoappendix consisting of the hernial sac. The remaining three had cecum and appendix sliding. Two of these had a paracecal ligament sliding into the hernial sac. No inflammatory adhesion with PPV wall or appendicitis was noted and none of these patients had blood perfusion disorder. Appendectomy was not done in any case. After division of each ligament and reduction of the cecal wall and appendix, the IIR was closed just distal to the viscera. A representative case is shown in Fig. 2.

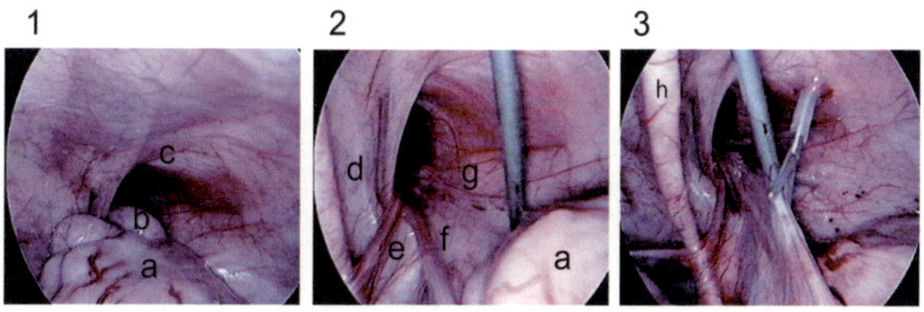

Figure 2. H.F., m, 7m, right indirect inguinal hernia. The cecum and appendix were found to slide into the hernial sac (1), which were easily pulled out remaining the paracecal ligament connecting to the vaginalis process (2). The paracecal ligament is being divided with an electro – scissors to make the cecum free in advance to closure of the PPV (3). Alphabets indicate; a, cecum; b, appendix; c, IIR; d, inferior epigastric vessels; e, spermatic cord; f, spermatic vessels; g, paracecal ligament; h, umbilical plica.

4.2. Bowel loops

Thirteen out of 14 patients were found in the LH group. Nine out of the 14 patients exhibited large hernia with long small intestinal loop slipping into the PPV without strangulation, of whom one boy underwent OH. These patients had been born prematurely and had widely open IIR and large hernial sac, and the loops were easily reduced. Four boys had strangulated loops, which were reduced by extracorporeal manual pressure under laparoscopic control with the assistance of internal pulling with a grasper. They revealed various degrees of perfusion disorder associated with petechiae, and viability was ascertained during the procedure (Fig. 3).

Their PPV orifices were found to be disproportionately small. In one girl, sliding ovary/adnexa appeared after reducing incarcerated bowel loops (Fig. 4). One boy had a sigmoid colon incarceration, in which no mesosigmoid sliding into the hernial sac was seen.

4.3. Omentum

In three patients, the preoperative diagnosis had been hydrocele. Seventeen out of 18 patients were included in the LH group. In six patients the omentum was found to slip into the PPV,

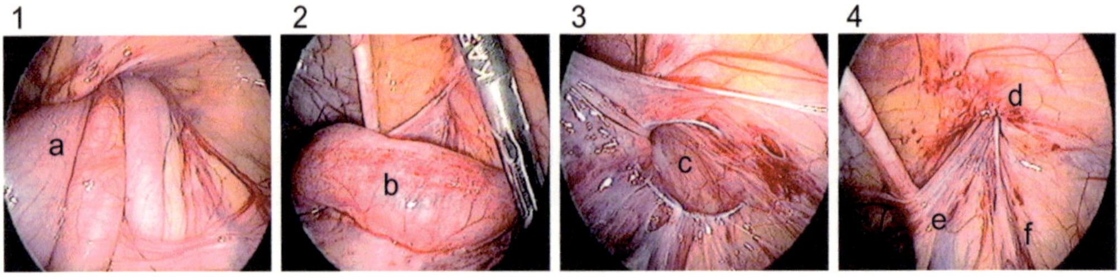

Figure 3. Y.H., m, 2y11m, right indirect inguinal hernia. Two loops of the small intestine were found to incarcerate into the hernial sac (1). The loops were pushed back into the peritoneal cavity from outside. Soon after released, the strangulated loop recovered leaving subserosal spotty hemorrhage (2). The suture has been placed around the IIR extraperitoneally, while the testicular vessels and spermatic cord were left intact (3). The end of the closure (4). Alphabets indicate; a, incarcerated bowel loop; b, subserosal petechiae; c, IIR encircled by extraperitoneally placed suture; d, closed IIR; e, spermatic cord; f, spermatic vessels.

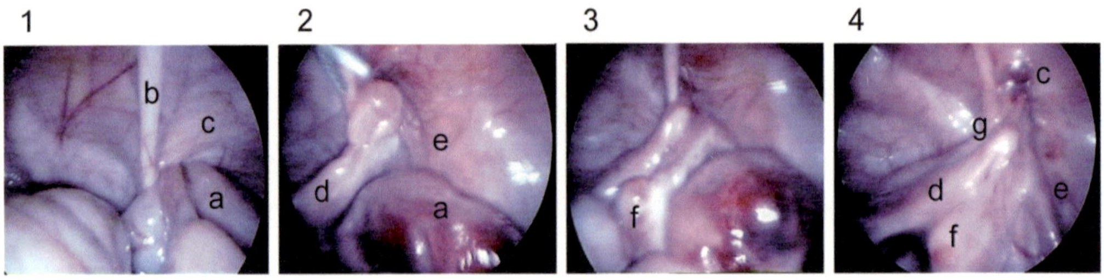

Figure 4. M.K., f, 8m, right indirect inguinal hernia. The incarcerated bowel loops are shown (1). The strangulated bowel loops have been released, while the ovary and adnexa remained in the sac. The bowel wall was partially associated with blood perfusion disorder with subserosal hemorrhage (2). In the next step, the ovary and adnexa were reducted. Spotty subserosal hemorrhages were seen also on the ovary (3). The IIR was closed distal to the U – turned Fallopian tube (4). Alphabets indicate; a, Incarcerated bowel loop; b, umbilical plica; c, IIR; d, uterus; e, ovarian vessels; f, ovary; g, U – turn point of Fallopian tube.

and was easily drawn out with a grasper. The remaining 12 patients had incarcerated omentum, where the tip of the omentum adhered to the bottom of the hernial sac. In two patients who underwent second – look herniorrhaphy for recurrence after previous OH, the omentum adhered to the operation scar in the recanalized PPV. In these cases, the omentum was reduced after dividing the tip with an electric scalpel (Fig. 5). Transient fluid accumulation in a distal sac with infarcted omental remnant occurred in one LH patient with incarceration of the omentum, which spontaneously disappeared during several days without sequela.

4.4. Ovary/adnexa

Twelve out of 53 patients were repaired by OH. There were four patients with uterine protrusion adding to ovary/adnexa sliding, where the LH findings showed a part of the uterus shared their wall with the hernial sac as a true sliding component. Fifteen patients had ovary/adnexa incarceration, of whom one had bilateral ovarian incarceration. Thirty – four patients had ovary/adnexa sliding, of whom two had bilateral ovarian sliding and one was associated with small bowel loop incarceration – the same case as described in "bowel loops". In all of

http://dx.doi.org/10.5772/58285

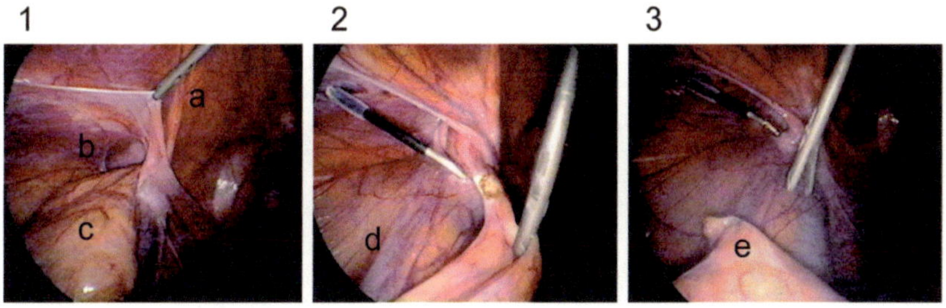

Figure 5. J.Y., m, 10y8m, left indirect inguinal hernia. The omentum had slipped into the vaginal process and its tip adhered to the bottom of the hernia sac (1). The omentum has been drawn out and is being cut off by an electrocautery at the adhesion point (2). The tip of the sliding omentum detached from the IIR (3). Alphabets indicate; a, umbilical plica; b, IIR; c, incarcerated omentum; d, spermatic vessels; e, detached omentum.

the patients, the uterus was found to be shifted to the affected side with shortened round ligament and the suspensory ligaments dislocated near the affected IIR (Fig. 6).

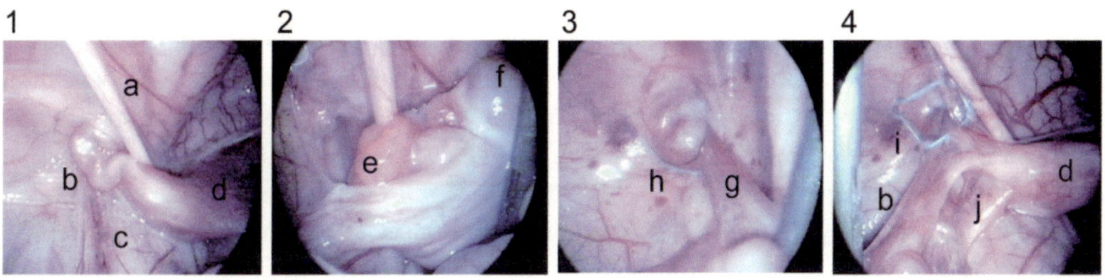

Figure 6. H.U., f, 2m, left indirect inguinal hernia. Sliding adnexa and the uterus shifting to the left side are shown (1). A scene showing released ovary and Fallopian tube (2). The ligamentum teres uteri stretched by a grasper with the sac inside out (3). The IIR encircled doubly (the first suture in a fashion of complete encircling and the second suture in interrupted one) distal to the running of the Fallopian tube (4). Alphabets indicate; a, umbilical plica; b, Fallopian tube running into the IIR; c, ovarian vessels; d, uterus shifted to the left; e, fimbria; f, ovary; g, round ligament; h, IIR encircled with first suture; i, IIR encircled with second suture; j, ovarian suspensory ligament.

In all of the patients with ovarian incarceration, the trapped ovary was twisted 240 to 1, 080 degrees (Fig. 7). The uterus – containing hernia patients, whose ages ranged from one to 3 months, were repaired with OH in one case, whose prolapsing viscera were pushed back into the peritoneal cavity and the IIR was closed with a modified Woolley, and LH in three, in whom after reducing the prolapsed organs into the peritoneal cavity, an extraperitoneal circuit suture was placed doubly just distal to the uterine and adnexa, without any complication. In LH, all ovaries and uteri with Fallopian tube were released ultimately without conversion to OH, although extracorporeal manual reduction was not so easy, and pulling of the adnexa with grasper was not advisable because of the risk of damage to the Fallopian tube. One girl with ovarian sliding suffered an accidental cut of the Fallopian tube during OH, which was anastomosed under microscopic surgery.

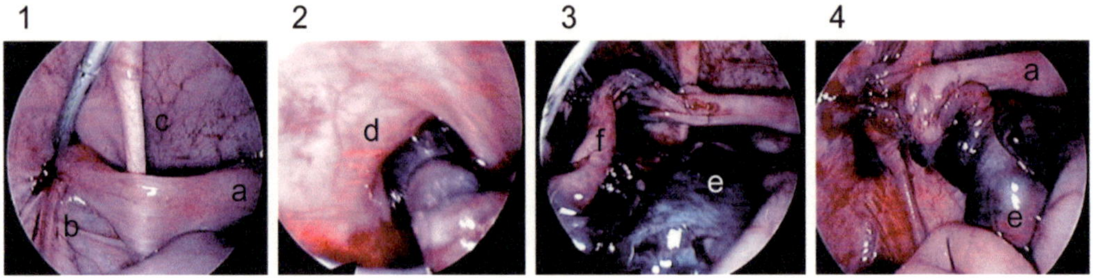

Figure 7. M.S., f, 6m, bilateral indirect inguinal hernia. Incarcerated adnexa with blood around the left IIR (1). The adnexa rotating 1, 080 degrees with strangulation (2). Released adnexa and ovary, which seemed necrotic (3). The IIR closed distal to the adnexa. Blood perfusion seems to begin returning (4). Alphabets indicate; a, uterus; b, ovarian vessels; c, umbilical plica; d, left IIR; e, ovary; f, Fallopian tube.

5. Discussion

Literature of the OH era has reported 12% incidence of incarceration/strangulation among 2, 764 pediatric hernias on admission [11]. Operation for incarcerated hernia in infants is particularly difficult because the sac is edematous and readily torn, rendering the testicular vessels and the vas vulnerable to trauma [9]. Repair of the hernial sac is not easy and inspection of the hernial sac contents after reduction is extremely difficult [5]. The complication rate was higher in cases of incarcerated hernia [1]. The overall complication rate after elective hernia repair was approximately 2%; this rose to 19% to 31% following operation for incarcerated hernia [3, 11]. Reported complications include infarction or atrophy of the testis or ovary, acquired undescended testis, vas transaction, bowel obstruction, intestinal necrosis, wound infection, and recurrent hernia [3, 4]. Nah et al. [4] stated, in comparing the outcomes of laparoscopic vs. open repair of incarcerated inguinal hernia, that the laparoscopic technique appeared safe, avoided the difficult dissection of edematous sac in the groin, allowed inspection of the reduced hernia content and permitted the repair of a cPPV if present.

Our series involved patients with S/IH in 5.1% of 1, 768 hernias, which showed lower incidence than Rowe's series [11], because our series contained only those patients who exhibited actual prolapse of the viscera into the hernial sac at the time of operation, and the patients whose S/IH had been reduced preoperatively was excluded. It has been stated that 45% to 84% of patients with incarcerated hernia on admission have successful manual reduction [3, 5].

Regarding the age distribution, 69% to 85% of the hernias occurred during the first year of life [3, 11]. In our series, 84.9% of patients were younger than one year of age. The reason why visceral protrusion tends to occur in young infants may be that in young infants the external inguinal ring is located so close to the IIR that the shortened inguinal canal becomes uncovered by musculature, and is thus vulnerable to increased intra – abdominal pressure [7]. In contrast, the average age of the patients with omental incarceration was six years. The reason here is that in the younger infants the omentum is still not well developed and needs several years to grow enough to reach the pelvic pouch.

Interestingly, Esposito et al. [5] reported that incarcerated hernia was more frequent in boys (65.2%) than in girls (27%), while Rowe et al. [11] mentioned slightly higher incidence in girls (17%) than in boys (12%). Our series showed significantly high incidence in girls. This may suggest higher rates of preoperative manual reduction in boys, while ovarian sliding or incarceration was not easy to be manually reduced. Actually, the incidence of I/SH in viscera other than ovary/adnexa was overwhelmingly high in boys (84.2%). In Rowe's series, 29% of incarcerated hernias in females required surgical reduction, compared with 17% in boys [11].

The proportion of OH and LH in ovary/adnexa S/IH was equal to the ratio in the WC, while those in the cecum/appendix, bowel loops and omentum groups were largely shifted to LH. This difference might be due to a bias of consideration of likelihood of operative difficulty in OH for incarcerated hernias. There was a tendency to attempt preoperative manual reduction more in the OH group among surgeons. The hernia content in 25 non – reducible hernias was reported as 60% in the adnexa/ovary, 36% in the bowel loops, 20% in the omentum group and 8% for the appendix group [5]. This was compatible with our series in terms of kinds and proportion of hernia content.

The presence of a vermiform appendix in the inguinal hernial sac is called Amyand's hernia, after the surgeon Claudius Amyand who reported the first case [12]. Most of these patients were male and the conditions of the herniated appendix were reported as normal, inflamed, or perforated. Some appendixes were found adhered to the inner hernial sac surface [13]. Preoperative diagnosis is said to be almost impossible, although ultrasound and computed tomography can help [14]. None of our patients underwent preoperative imaging, but intraoperative diagnosis was quite easy. Our series did not include the inflamed appendix. Fifty percent of our patients had mesoappendix or paracecal ligament sliding into the hernial sac. We are not aware of any paper that has reported cecal S/IH.

Bowel loop incarceration is the most serious condition in male infants. The conventional treatment is trial of manual reduction and to delay of surgical repair in order to reduce the surgical risk in a traumatized edematous anatomy [6]. In our OH group, patients were managed in this way, while in the LH group a too – strong manual reduction was avoided to prohibit the damage to the strangulated loop, because the loop should be controlled under laparoscopic direct vision. Our patients consisted of two groups: infants with a widely open IIR and large hernial sac, in which many bowel loops were contained but easily reduced by external manual compression under intraperitoneal direct inspection, and infants with narrow IIR and sac containing loops with various degrees of perfusion disorder. In the latter cases, difficulty was encountered at the IIR in reducing the bowel, although a combined technique of external manual pressure and internal pulling by forceps was ultimately successful. Vigorous grasping and pulling of the bowel loop induced damage to the intestinal serosa. In these cases, the dilation of the IIR with a retractor or adding of an incision to the internal oblique muscle would be recommended in OH [9].

Omental incarceration causing hydrocele has been reported [15]. Here, the average age was 4.5 years, a little bit lower than our series. In our series, three of 18 patients had been preoperatively diagnosed as hydrocele. In omental incarceration, 67% of patients had their omental tip adhered to the wall of the PPV. This might be an outcome of the role of the omentum, which moves to the damaged part of the intraperitoneal organs, for example with inflammation, wall defect or hernia. The hernial sac containing omentum closely mimicked the soft hydrocele on palpation, especially when it was not reducible due to adhesion with the bottom of the hernial sac. The groin mass was soft, not reducible without pain or tenderness.

The advantage of LH was highlighted in female infants with sliding or incarcerated ovary/adnexa. Articles have reported that 15 – 22.4% of the inguinal hernias in female children are sliding hernias, and that the most frequently sliding organ is the ovary, followed by the Fallopian tubes [16]. Drawbacks associated with the reproductive system are a hidden but not a negligible problem. Fallopian tube obstruction or displacement of the ovary and Fallopian tube in the retroperitoneal space in a woman with a history of childhood inguinal herniorrhaphy has been reported as the cause of infertility [17 – 19]. We had an episode of injury to the Fallopian tube during OH for ovarian sliding hernia. OH requires the traction of the round ligament from the outside so as to obtain a good visual field and achieve high ligation [20], resulting in the remainder of the U – turned Fallopian tube in the hernial sac as acting a sliding component after reducing the ovary. Careless handling of the neck of the hernial sac can induce cutting or ligation of the Fallopian tube. Especially in female infant S/IH, the round ligament is shortened and the ovarian suspensory ligament is ventrally dislocated, facilitating the inducing of tubal occlusion as a postoperative complication [21].

Strangulation of irreducible ovaries has been reported with an incidence of 2% to 33% [22]. The incidence in our series was 28.3%. The laparoscopic findings suggested that the ovaries went into the inguinal canal through narrow IIR, twisting themselves. Uterus – containing inguinal hernia is an extremely rare condition, with 0.23% incidence [23]. The uterus may be free within the sac, adherent to the wall by adhesions or a true sliding component. [23]. In the treatment of ovary/adnexa I/SH including uterine sliding by LH, after reducing the prolapsing organs, the IIR was encircled by a suture proximal to the IIR level, placing all the surrounding viscera out of the IIR, without any special resources like OH.

In the international literature, a small number of studies have been published on laparoscopic treatment of incarcerated or sliding inguinal hernia, in particular a comparative study between laparoscopy and open surgery. Nah et al. [4] emphasized the superiority of LH in his comparative study from the viewpoint of operative complication, stating that LH presented a lower complication rate (4%) compared to OH (14%). Difficulties in identifying the correct relation of the anatomic structures, occasionally encountered in open procedures, practically almost never occur with the laparoscopic approach [6]. The advantages of the laparoscopic approach have been reported as follows: a lower incidence of complications, technically easy, all edematous tissue surgically bypassed, the cord structures not touched, reduction under direct visual control, inspection of the incarcerated organ at the end of procedure, simultaneous repair of cPPV if present [4, 5].

In our series, all the procedures with LH were completed without conversions, without serious complication and without recurrence, although all the procedures were successful also in OH, except for one Fallopian tube accident. The fact that mean operation time in the OH group exceeded the time of bilateral OH in the WC, while the time of the LH group was equal to the WC and shorter than for the OH group, indicates the technical easiness of LH. In traditional open repair of I/SH, preoperative diagnostic imaging such as ultrasound and computed tomography have been recommended for differentiating the hernial content [14, 24, 25]. The laparoscopic approach could free patients from these preoperative examinations, because intraperitoneal inspection resolved every ambiguousness around the IIR and in the hernial sac.

6. Conclusion

The advantages of laparoscopic approach are that it is technically simple with short operation time, and that there is the possibility for direct inspection of incarcerated/sliding viscera before and after resolution, as well as closure of internal inguinal rings, avoiding injury to the reproductive systems. This comparative study has validated the feasibility of the laparoscopic approach, suggesting that this approach should be allowed to take the place of the gold standard in treatment of children with incarcerated/sliding indirect inguinal hernia.

Author details

Masao Endo*, Michinobu Ohno, Fumiko Yoshida, Miwako Nakano, Toshihiko Watanabe and Etsuji Ukiyama

*Address all correspondence to: emta@mxr.mesh.ne.jp

Department of Pediatric Surgery, Saitama City Hospital, Mimuro, Midori – ku, Saitama – shi, Japan

References

[1] Erdogan D, Karaman I, Aslan MK, Karaman A, Cavusoglu YH. Analysis of 3, 776 Pediatric Inguinal Hernia and Hydrocele Cases in a Tertiary Center. J Pediatr Surg 2013; 48(8) 1767 – 1772.

[2] Niedzielski J, KrlR, Gawlowska A. Could Incarceration of Inguinal Hernia in Children be Prevented? Med Sci Monit 2003; 9(1) CR16 – 18.

[3] Stylianos S, Jacir NN, Harris BH. Incarceration of Inguinal Hernia in Infants prior to Elective Repair. J Pediatr Surg 1993;28(4) 582 – 583.

[4] Nah SA, Giacomello L, Eaton S, de Coppi P, Curry JI, Drake DP, Kiely EM, Pierro A. Surgical Repair of Incarcerated Inguinal Hernia in Children: Laparoscopic or Open? Eur J Pediatr Surg 2011; 21(1) 8 – 11.

[5] Esposito C, Turial S, Alicchio F, Enders J, Castagnetti M, Krause K, Settimi A, Schier F. Laparoscopic Repair of Incarcerated Inguinal Hernia. A Safe and Effective Procedure to Adopt in Children. Hernia 2013;17(2) 235 – 239.

[6] Kaya M, Huckstedt T, Schier F. Laparoscopic Approach to Incarcerated Inguinal Hernia in Children. J Pediatr Surg 2006;41(3) 567 – 569.

[7] Endo M, Watanabe T, Nakano M, Yoshida F, Ukiyama E. Laparoscopic Completely Extraperitoneal Repair of Inguinal Hernia in Children: A Single Institute Experience with 1, 257 Repairs Compared with Cut – down Herniorrhaphy. Surg Endosc 2009;23(8) 1706 – 1712.

[8] Endo M, Ukiyama E. Laparoscopic Closure of Patent Processus Vaginalis in Girls with Inguinal Hernia Using a Specially Devised Suture Needle. Ped Endosurg Innov Techn 2001; 5:187 – 191.

[9] Rowe MI, Lloyd DA. Inguinal Hernia. In: Welch KJ, Randolph JG, Ravitch MM, O'Neil JA Jr, Rowe MI. (eds.) Pediatric Surgery 4thED. Chicago, London: Year Book Medical Publishers; 1986. p779 – 793.

[10] Woolley MM. Inguinal hernia. In: Pediatric Surgery 3rdED. Chicago: Year Book Medical Publishers; 1979. p815.

[11] Rowe MI, Clatworthy HW. Incarcerated and Strangulated Hernias in Children. A Statistical Study of High – risk Factors. Arch Surg 1970;101: 136 – 139.

[12] Lombardo V, Pavone G. Intraoperative Finding of Amyand's Hernia in a Recurrent Inguinal Hernia. Report of a Case. Ann Ital Chir 2013; 84: 583 – 584.

[13] Okur MH, Karacay S, Uygun I, Topcu K, Ozturk H. Amyand's Hernias in Childhood (a Report on 21 Patients): a Single – center Experience. Pediatr Surg Int 2013; 29(6) 571 – 574.

[14] Michalinos A, Moris D, Vernadakis S. Amyand's Hernia: a Review. Am J Surg 2013, pii: S0002 – 9610(13)00646 – 6. Doi: 10.1016/j.amjsurg.2013.07043. [Epub ahead of print]

[15] Kapisiz A, Karabulut R, Turkyilmaz Z, Sonmez K, Basaklar AC. Omental Incarceration may Cause Hydrocele and this Hydrocele Confused Simple or Scrotal Hydrocele. Hernia 2011; 15(1) 43 – 45.

[16] Turk E, Fescekoglu OR, Acari C, Karaca F, Bilen CM, Edirne Y, Karakaya E. Sliding Hernia in Female Children. Acta Chir Belg 2013; 113(4) 281 – 284.

[17] Swanson JA, Chapler FK. Infertility as a Consequence of Bilateral Inguinal Herniorrhaphies. Fertil Steril 1977; 28(10) 1118 – 1120.

[18] Cam C, Celik C, Sancak A, Iskender C, Karateke A. Inguinal Herniorrhaphy in Childhood may Result in Tubal Damage and Future Infertility. Arch Gynecol Obstet 2009; 279(2) 175 – 176.

[19] Gueth U, Renner R, Egelhof T, Singer G, Holzgreve W, Mayr J. Retroperitoneal Displacement of Ovary and Fallopian Tube: a Complication of Surgical Management of Incarcerated Inguinal Hernia in Female Infants. J Pediatr Surg; 2007; 42(5) E33 – 35.

[20] Endo M, Ohno M, Yoshida F, Nakano M, Watanabe T, Ukiyama E. Laparoscopic Hernia Repair and its Validation by Second – look Inspection to Internal Inguinal Rings in Children with Patent Processus Vaginalis. In: Meinhold – Heerlein I. (ed.) Laparoscopy – An Interdisciplinary Approach. Rijeka: InTech; 2011. p133 – 146. Available from http://www.intechopen.com

[21] Hirabayashi T, Sakoda A, Kawano T. Ventrally Dislocated Attachment of the Ovarian Suspensory Ligament, a Risk Factor for Tubal Occlusion as a Postoperative Complication of Inguinal Hernia Repair: Efficacy of Laparoscopic Inguinal Hernia Repair for Preventing Tubal Damage. Pediat Surg Int 2012; 28(11) 1089 – 1094.

[22] Boley SJ, Cahn D, Lauer T, Weinberg G, Kleinhaus S. The Irreducible Ovary: a True Emergency. J Pediatr Surg 1991; 26(9) 1035 – 1038.

[23] Akillioglu L, Kaymakci A, Akkoyun I, Guven S, Yucesan S, Hicsonmez A. Inguinal Hernias Containing the Uterus; a Case Series of 7 Female Children. J Pediatr Surg 2013; 48(10) 2157 – 2159.

[24] Narci A, Korkmaz M, Albyrak R, Sozubir S, Guvenc BH, Koken R, Demir T, Dogru O. Preoperative Sonography of Nonreducible Inguinal Masses in Girls. J Clin Ultrasound 2008; 36(7) 409 – 412.

[25] Akfirat M, Kazez A, Serhatilioglu S. Preoperative Sonographic Diagnosis of Sliding Appendicial Inguinal Hernia. J Clin Ultrasound 1999; 27(3) 156 – 158.

Laparoscopic Inguinal Preperitoneal Injection (LIPI) — Novel Experimental Technique for Inguinal Hernia Repair in Children

Yury Kozlov, Vladimir Novozhilov,
Vitaly Kovalev and Pavel Krasnov

Additional information is available at the end of the chapter

http://dx.doi.org/10.5772/57159

1. Introduction

Inguinal hernia repair is the most common procedure in pediatric surgery. Suture techniques for laparoscopic inguinal hernia repair in children are easy to perform and popular with a low recurrence rate. The aim of this study was to evaluate the effect of laparoscopic preperitoneal injection of 3-dimensional gel on closing of the inguinal hernia sac (IHS) in laboratory animals. We performed peritoneoscopy by 12 male Chinchilla rabbits weighing 1200 to 1400 g. Endoscope was introduced in abdominal cavity and bilateral deep inguinal rings were identified. The needle Tuohy with the injectable polymeric bulking agent DAM+ (3-Dimensional Polyacrylamide gel with Ions of Silver "Argiform", Bioform®) was introduced preperitoneally. The implant was then injected across the entire orifice of the deep inguinal rings and draped over the cord structures. After completion of bilateral repairs, the rabbits were extubated and observed in animal laboratory. Then the second laparoscopy was performed 6 months after and the deep inguinal rings were inspected. At second laparoscopy no reopening to the entire orifice of the deep inguinal rings were noted. Accurate placement the polymeric agent and adequate coverage of the vas deferens was accomplished in all animals. This scientific report demonstrates that the biopolymeric implant gives good postoperative results and a stable trend of closing IHS in long-term follow-up. We hope that the injectable polymeric bulking agents can be used for treatment of inguinal hernias at pediatric patients after additional animal and human researches.

Inguinal hernia is the most frequent diagnosis in pediatric surgery. Familiarity with embryology is necessary to understand the inguinal abnormalities. During fetal life, the descent of the testis into the inguinal canal and scrotum brings a small pouch of peritoneum alongside. This peritoneal extension is the processus vaginalis. In females, the formation of the labia has the same peritoneal remnant, referred to as the canal of Nuck. The peritoneal canals are obliterated in up to 95–98% of fetuses before birth. Failure of this peritoneal fusion results in a spectrum of abnormalities. The degree of fusion failure results in either a hydrocele or a hernia [1, 2]. There are two types of inguinal hernia: direct, where the abdominal musculature is weak and visceral contents protrude through the wall of the inguinal canal and exit via the superficial inguinal ring, and indirect inguinal hernia, where visceral contents pass into the patent processus vaginalis (PPV) via an open deep inguinal ring and exit via the superficial inguinal rings. The latter is the most common finding in children.

Inguinal hernia in children can be repaired through either an open or laparoscopic technique. In 1995, Shcheben'kov [3] first reported on laparoscopic inguinal hernia repair in pediatric patients. Since that time, laparoscopic ligation of inguinal hernias has been performed in many institutions with a variety of methods of suturing of open inguinal rings.

The laparoscopic approach can be performed either transperitoneally or through a preperitoneal approach with transperitoneal visualization. The transperitoneal method incorporates a telescope through an umbilical port, allowing direct visualization of the deep inguinal rings, followed by the controlled passage of instruments either with or without the assistance of trocars. The deep ring is then closed with either an absorbable or nonabsorbable suture either as purse string or similar (Fig.1).

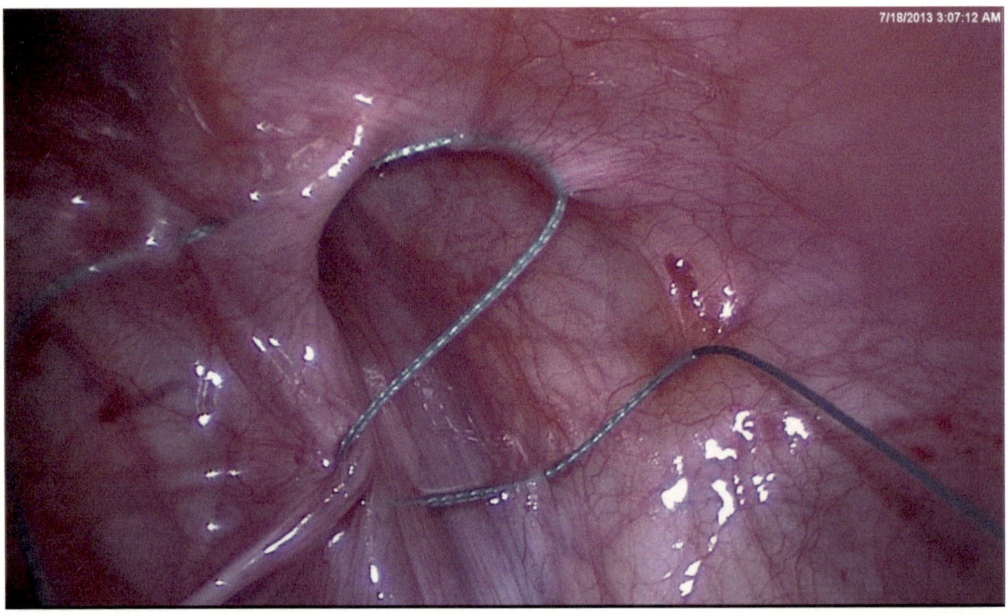

Figure 1. Transperitoneal ligation of the internal inguinal ring by Schier (Z-suture)

http://dx.doi.org/10.5772/57159

Since the description of extraperitoneally ligation of the internal inguinal ring by Takehara [4] and Ozdegiz [5], the treatment of inguinal hernias at children was transformed to «story of needles and hooks». A small hook or Tuohy needle, loaded with a suture, is passed around the deep ring after making a small inguinal skin incision. The passage of the suture is observed via an endoscope at the umbilicus (Fig.2). The ligature is then brought extracorporally and tied, thus closing the hernial orifice. The transabdominal extraperitoneal repair has some support for a lower recurrence rate, when compared to the traditional open procedure. A slightly higher recurrence rate appears to exist when comparing the transperitoneal to the extraperitoneal and open repair. The advantages of a reduced injury to the vas and vessels, a reduction in testicular atrophy, and improved cosmesis are not supported by current levels of evidence.

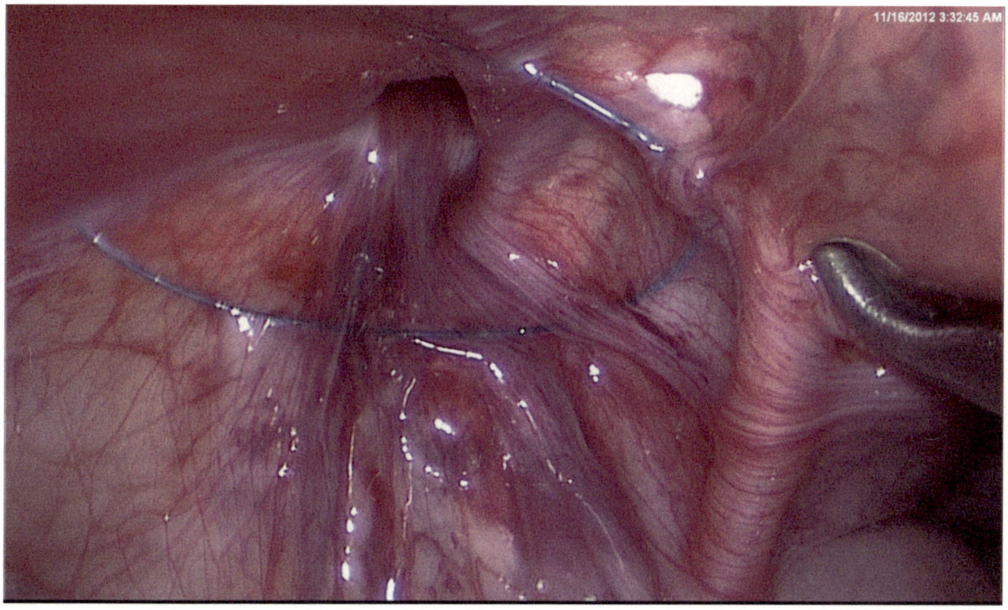

Figure 2. Preperitoneal ligation of the internal inguinal ring by Ozdegiz

Complications are rare following surgery for hernia or hydrocele. Injury to the vas deferens during inguinal or hydrocele repair is a potential risk [6] with treatment requiring microsurgical repair. Visceral injury during laparoscopic repair is very rare and can be treated either by open or laparoscopic surgery. Injury to the genitofemoral nerve, resulting in chronic pain, is a rare occurrence [7]. Testicular ascent following inguinal tissue contracture is another possible long-term problem as well as testicular atrophy, though the latter is associated usually with preoperative incarceration.

The surgical principal in laparoscopic repair in children is to close the inguinal hernia sac (IHS) at its neck as in the open repair. Different techniques of laparoscopic hernia repair have been developed, but there are two basic approaches – a purely intracorporeal [8-11] ligation and laparoscopic-assisted extracorporeal ligation [4, 5]. Therefore, further development in minimal access surgery for pediatric inguinal hernia is to decrease the number and size of skin incisions. With a trend toward increasing use of extracorporeal knotting and decreasing use of working ports and endoscopic instruments, single-port endoscopy-assisted percutaneous extraperitoneal closure with variable devices is the attainment.

Laparoscopic approach to inguinal hernia in children has become an alternative to the conventional open procedure. Advantages of endoscopic repairs include the ability to evaluate the contralateral side, avoidance of access trauma to the vas deferens and gonadal vessels, iatrogenic cryptorchidism, shorter operative time, less postoperative pain and length of hospital stay. According to the literature, open herniorhaphy in children has been reported to have recurrence rate of 0.8% to 3.8% and postoperative contralateral hernia rates up to 30% [12, 17]. Recurrence rates in laparoscopic approach has ranged from 0.7% to 4.3% [13, 14].

There are some technical limitations, although modifications on laparoscopic surgery continue to be refined. The known limitations of the laparoscopic surgery are as follows - the necessity for intra-abdominal skills, such as intracorporeal suturing, knot tying, and manipulation of the suture on a needle, high operating costs and cardiorespiratory changes by pneumoperitoneum. In fact, compared with open herniotomy, laparoscopic approach did not take any superiority in cosmesis. Conversely, the procedure was thought not to be a minimally invasive surgery because of the necessity of multiple skin incisions and pneumoperitoneum during operation.

2. Polymers in inguinal surgery

Laparoscopic inguinal hernia repair involves less dissection of the abdominal wall and spermatic cord structures, so the risk for complications may be lower, but some kind of suture (ie, z-suture, n-suture, purse string suture, and extraperitoneal closure) must be used. Placing his sutures correctly is difficult, and there is a considerable learning curve involved, especially in premature, because of the extremely limited operative field. In contrast, deep inguinal ring does not require surgical ligation, and can be closed using injected tissue adhesive.

Laparoscopic hernia surgery continues to evolve with new polymeric products allowing surgeons multiple choices in treating their patients. In 2004 Miyano G. et al. [15], published experimental work with injection of 2-octyl-cyanoacrylate (Dermabond®) into right IHS under laparoscopic control. Herniography results showed no flow of gastrografin solution into treated inguinal hernia sac in rats. Histologic examination in the treated HIS demonstrated localized mild inflammation, and foreign body giant cells were observed around the Dermabond®. The spermatic vessels, vas deferens, and testes were normal. All testes had large numbers of normal sperm. This technique is innovative concept for the treatment of inguinal hernia because it uses tissue adhesives to close hernia sac. This approach eliminates dissection of the spermatic cord and ligation of the IHS, thus virtually completely lowering the risks of injuries. Later, in 2005, the same group of authors published paper comparing several types of tissue adhesives in the treatment of inguinal hernia [16]. This experimental work has shown high efficiency of Dermabond® for closing IHS. Explanation of this efficiency is that this tissue agent is not absorbable. The other tissue adhesives are all absorbable, and may have become ineffective within months. Comparing different tissue adhesives Kato Y. et al. have shown that laparoscopic injection of 2-octyl-cyanoacrylate (Dermabond®) was highly effective for closing the orifice of the IHS [16]. Following study [17] demonstrates that fibrin glue and cyanoacrylate are better tolerated than sutures by patients, and that the glues lead to better results during initial follow-up and a better trend in long-term data. The glues were recommended for use in adults for mesh fixation of tension-free inguinal repair.

3. Polyacrylamides in surgery

Injectable soft tissue fillers play an important role in cosmetic and reconstructive surgery. Since the acceptance of collagen as a filler, new reabsorbable and non-absorbable implants have appeared with varying degrees of success. Today, as we know more about products and their potential complications, a more accurate treatment plan can be arranged for the patient. The ideal desired characteristics for a soft tissue filler are that they must be safe, biocompatible, easy to inject, long lasting effect, and not provoke any complications. Nonbiodegradable fillers must give a definitive correction. The advantage of these products is longevity. One of these products is polyacrylamide. The chemical properties of polyacrylamide gel with a high proportion of water cause fewer foreign body reactions. The capsule gets thicker with fibroblasts and macrophage accumulation. This product is the first choice for facial soft tissue augmentation, such a cheek, chin, or mandibular augmentation. Polyacrylamide adds volume to the subcutaneous tissue, thereby restoring of augmentic facial and body contours. It is also used for lip augmentation, nasolabial folds, perioral wrinkles, glabellar frown lines, and depressed mouth corners. This product must be injected deeply in the subcutaneous tissues. Polyacrylamide implantation is considered permanent. It cannot be reabsorbed into the body. Hydrophilic polyacrylamide gels are non-toxic, non-sensitizing, non-mutagenic, biocompatible and chemically stable. After injection the water content is absorbed by the body whilst the gel becomes encapsulated. It remains soft and pliable like the body's own tissue.

In our experimental study we proposed the laparoscopic preperitoneal injection of 3-Dimensional gel (DAM+™) on closing the orifice of the IHS in laboratory animals. This polymer is injectable hydrophilic polyacrylamide gel with 0.03% residual unpolymerized acrylamide monomer. It is manufactured by Bioform in Russia. This product is the second generation polyacrylamide gel comprised of 95% polyacrylamide and 5% water, it is also manufactured using a silver ion process to help repel bacteria. It comes in sterile syringe with a needle of 25Gx1½ (Fig.3). Prepacked and tested for microbiological cleanness the gel DAM+ is then sterilized in an autoclave chamber and tested for sterility. The 3-D polymeric gel is the most physiological and the safest implant out of the rest existing implants. Its structure and properties respond in the best way to the inner space of the human body. It contains silver, which creates unfavorable medium against bacterial invasion and development of pathogenic microbiological flora. This filling agent is inert, does not react to the previously injected gels, admits possibility of its multiple injections into the same anatomical region in the case it has been not enough injected or applied in stage-by-stage corrections. DAM+ can be injected through thin needles, hence it causes minimal traumas. It is very important that it does not cause an inflammation, nor any allergy or non-compatibility with the tissues thanks to absence in it of initiators of immune reactions. During long-term localization within the injection zone, DAM+ does not exert any inflammatory reactions. When injected correctly, it does not migrate from the injection zone.

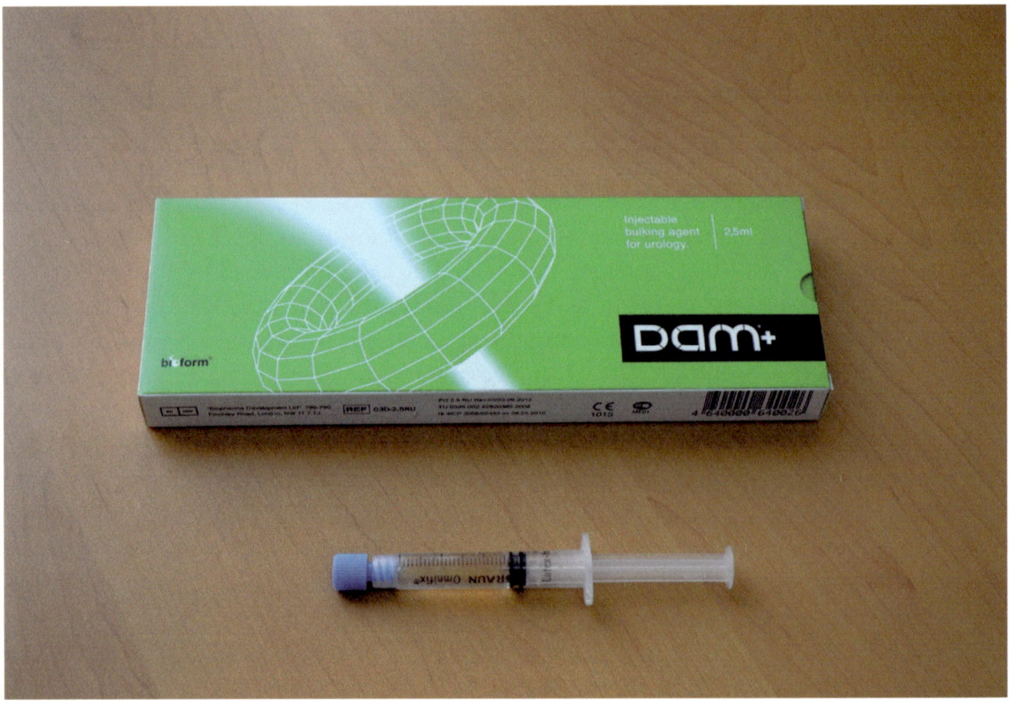

Figure 3. Polyacrylamide gel DAM+ in packing

This agent is used in clinical practice for endoprothesis of the soft tissues by increases of their volume. Polyacrylamide in fact has been used for decades in the preparation of soft contact lenses. Besides, the toxicity of polyacrylamide has been studied for more than 30 years. Research indicates that polyacrylamide is non toxic and practically non biodegradable. DAM + is absolutely safe because of the presence of silver ions, known for their antibacterial properties. There are also no allergy issues with this gel. There are some articles with good results of using this gel in bronchial surgery for endoscopic treatment of bronchial fistulas and prophylaxis, treatment of primary insufficiency of bronchial stump after pneumonectomy [18, 19] and in endoscopic treatment of vesico-ureteral reflux in children [20]. Safety of the hydrophilic gel DAM+ has been repeatedly confirmed by its pre-clinical tests on animals, also by its experimental clinical application [21]. In this experimental study it was shown that polyacrylamide gel had low reactivity with surrounding tissue. Ions of silver contribute to this low reactivity and reduce the risks of local inflammation. The histological examination has shown development of good capsule with macrophageal infiltration, marked vascularity and absence of any signs of local inflammation. In microscopic research 1 month after the operation, the implanted material remained located in the subcutaneous cellular tissue in the form of grid structures of fibrous character. There was a round cell reaction observed with excess of macrophage elements. Three months after the implantation, the histopathologic feature got changed. Thin polymer taenias penetrating into the tissue had developed in all directions from the main conglomerate of the implanted material. That phenomenon was explained by the fact that a conjunctive capsule began its formation. Within the connective tissue, not far from the implanted material, vessels were seen enlarged plethoric blood vessels. After six months, around the implanted material revealed a connective tissue infiltrated with macrophages and other round cell elements and marked the development of the capsule. In some areas around the implanted material observed a mature connective capsule isolating the polymer from the surrounding tissues. The main components of that capsule were collagen fibers and mature fusiform fibroblasts between them. Reaction of the blood system remained expressive, some vessels were enlarged and plethoric.

4. Experimental technique of laparoscopic inguinal preperitoneal injection (LIPI)

Minimally invasive surgery has become more frequent in children in the last decade. These techniques require special training because of the low incidence of many surgical diseases in children, and the skills needed are difficult to acquire. For this purpose, several training models have been used, including endotraining boxes, animals, and, more recently, virtual reality. The smaller size of pediatric patients requires not only adequate endoscopic instruments but also an appropriate animal model for teaching and training pediatric minimally invasive surgery.

The most commonly used animals are pigs, which are good models only for big children and adolescents; furthermore, they are expensive and hard to obtain. Rabbits are commonly used in experimental medicine, easy to obtain, very similar in weight to a newborn, and less expensive than pigs. Reports of laparoscopy performed for experimental laparoscopic surgical procedures in rabbits, including the gasless model [22], and other procedures, mainly in gynecology [23-26], prompted us to choose the adult rabbit as our training model for treatment of inguinal hernia. The naturally opened inguinal duct in rabbits resembles the human inguinal hernia with peritoneal fold. Because of inguinal canal of rabbits remains open and patent throughout life and the internal inguinal ring is also open and wide, they are chosen for laboratory study. Simple cohort of twelve male Chinchilla rabbits weighing 1200 to 1400 g was used as subjects. All animals had unrestricted access to food and water pre- and postoperatively. Experimental work was done according to the "Hospital experimental work state" and was approved by hospital ethical committee.

This work was developed at the Experimental Surgery Center of the Institute of Surgery Irkutsk, Russia. A 5-mm 30-degree endoscope without additional laparoscopic instruments was used. All procedures were recorded on hard disk of the videohub. All animals were placed supine and laparoscopy was done under general anesthesia. Acepromazine (0,25 mg/kg), midazolam (1 mg/kg) and meperidine (5 mg/kg) were administrated intramuscularly as premedication. The induction to general anesthesia was performed with Isoflurane 5%, using a tracheal tube, and maintained with Isoflurane 3-4% under manual ventilation. The animals were positioned supine over a surgical table and kept in place with elastic bands. The abdomen had previously been shaved. All needle movements are performed from outside the body cavity under camera control. To choose the location for the needle puncture, the position of the internal inguinal ring is assessed by pressing the inguinal region from the outside with the tip of a Pean forceps (Fig.4).

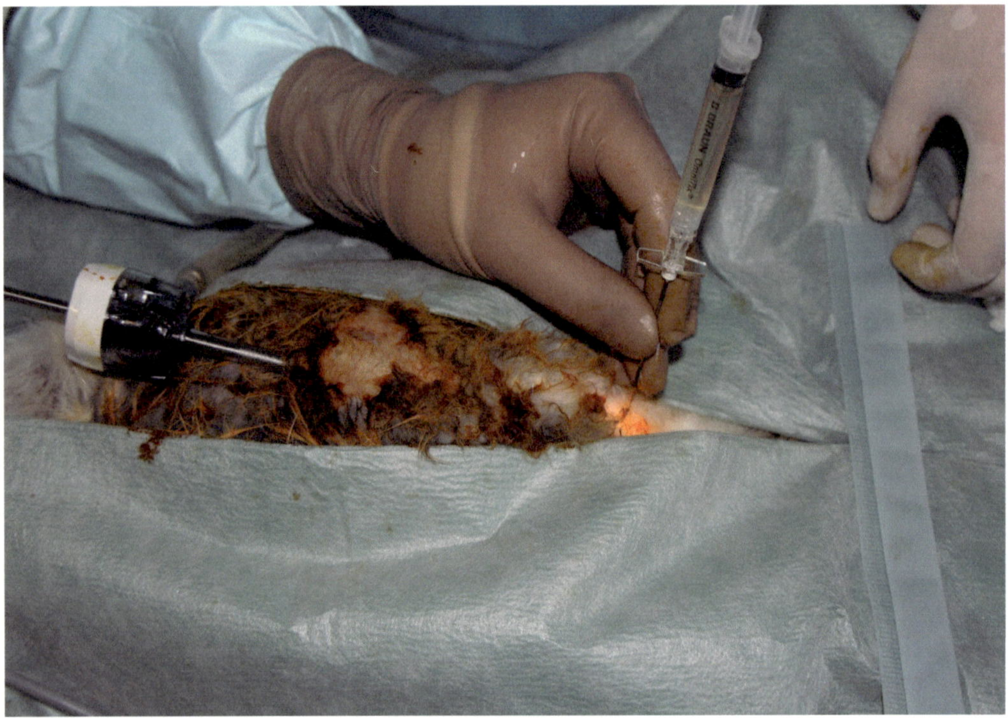

Figure 4. Position telescope and Tuohy needle during laparoscopic inguinal preperitoneal injection (LIPI)

At the beginning of procedure was performed the inspection of deep inguinal rings and cord structures (Fig.5). The Tuohy needle with injectable polymeric bulking agent DAM+™ (3-Dimensional polyacrylamide gel with ions of silver "Argiform", Bioform®) was introduced preperitoneally (Fig.6). The 2.0 ml of implant was then injected across the entire orifice of the internal inguinal rings (Fig.7) and draped over the cord structures (Fig.8). Mean operative time ranged from 10 to 12 minutes for bilateral hernia repair. Time required to inject the DAM+™ was less than 1 minute Postoperative recovery was rapid and all animals returned to their normal activity after the procedure.

http://dx.doi.org/10.5772/57159

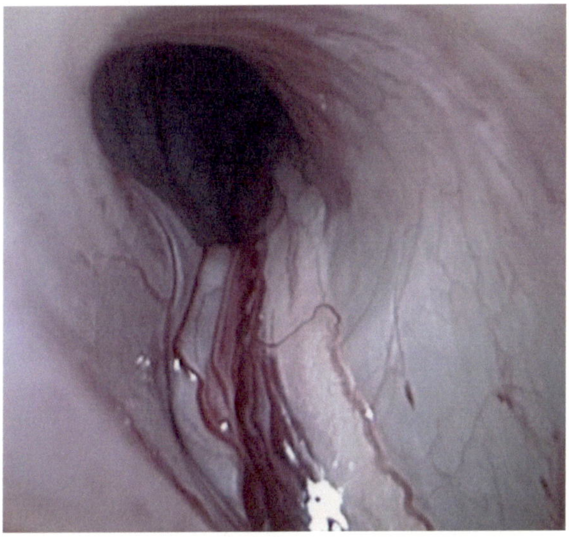

Figure 5. Laparoscopic view on the orifice of the inguinal hernia sac (IHS), the spermatic cord and vas deferens in rabbit

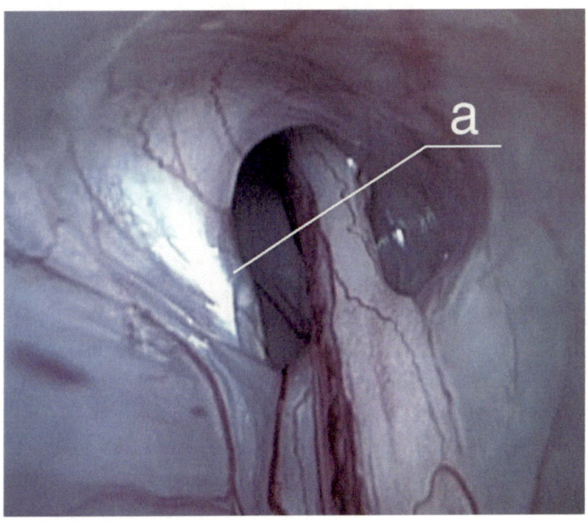

Figure 6. Tip of the Tuohy needle (a) before the gels implantation

After injection of the bulking agent and closing of the orifice of the IHS, the rabbits were extubated and observed in animal laboratory. Second laparoscopy was performed six month later using the same technique. At the second procedure the integrity of the closed internal inguinal rings and the presence of ring abscess, peritonitis and adhesions were recorded. At second laparoscopy integrity of the closed internal inguinal ring was present. No opening of the rings was observed. Accurate placement of the polymeric agent and adequate coverage of

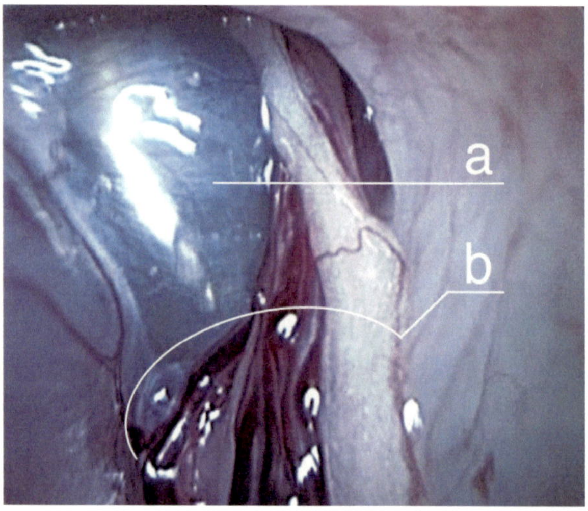

Figure 7. Tip of the Tuohy needle (a) after the gels implantation (b – spermatic cord)

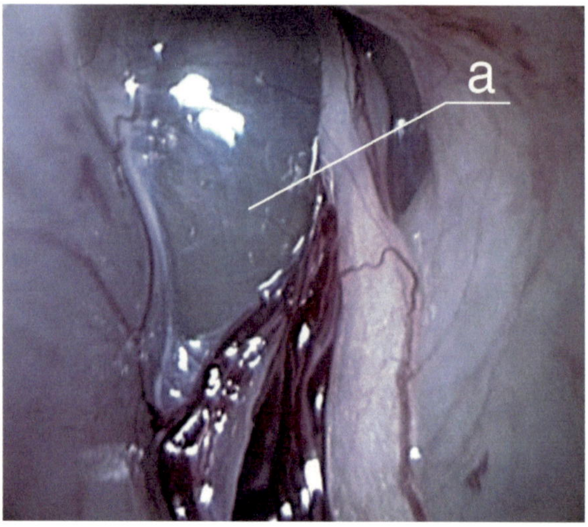

Figure 8. View of the inguinal hernia sac after LIPI procedure with preperitoneal placement of the polymeric agent (a)

the vas deferens were accomplished in all animals. Adhesions between the closed orifice of the IHS and the small bowel were absent in all rabbits. There were no signs of peritonitis and abscess formation.

In the current study, histologic examination clearly showed that mild inflammation was localized within the IHS only adjacent to the gel and there were no histopathologic changes detected around the vas deferens and spermatic vessels. Our results has shown that after six months of DAM+™ injection closing of internal inguinal ring was observed with no reopening in all cases. This technique is simple, safe, and does not require any laparoscopic skills. Our method is highly successful, but in preparation for its use clinically, we must perform a particular studies requiring investigation local tissue reaction and long-term follow-up after the gel injection. In addition, we have concerns about hernia recurrence because polyacrylamide gel may lose its volume effect. Such research will confirm if there are any detrimental sequelae associated with this technique.

5. Application in the future

Progress in pediatric surgery and anesthesia has reduced the risk of the procedure of the hernioraphy so that in most centers it is performed as a day surgery. Further development in minimal access surgery for pediatric inguinal hernia is to decrease the number and size of skin incisions. With a trend toward increasing use of extracorporeal knotting and decreasing use of working ports and endoscopic instruments, laparoscopic inguinal preperitoneal injection (LIPI) of 3-D gel may be the attainment. We develop a modified technique of non-operative treatment of the inguinal hernia in children and we assume that gel injection in preperitoneale space can be performed under ultrasound visualization without laparoscopic control.

A technology of ultrasound guided nerve block in infants undergoing inguinal hernioraphy gained special popularity in pediatric anesthesia recently. The ilioinguinal/iliohypogastric nerve block is a popular regional anesthetic technique for postoperative pain relief after inguinal surgery in children [27, 28]. It is not easily to perform because the peritoneal cavity is just millimeters from the ilioinguinal and iliohypogastric nerves in small children. Needle placement and spread of local anesthetic is easily seen with high-resolution ultrasonography. Using ultrasound guidance, greater success can be achieved by more accurate placement of reduced volumes of local anesthetics closer to the targeted nerves.

We can transfer this technique and make similar procedure for a gel injection at pediatric patients with inguinal hernia. The idea consists in the following. Before placement of the 3-D polyacrylamide gel an initial ultrasound exploration of the area of the proposed injection site is performed by an experienced ultrasonographer using a stationary or transportable ultrasound unit and a 5–10 MHz linear probe with an active area of 20-30 mm. Inguinal masses in children must be carefully evaluated. The proposed site of injection will be then prepared with chlorhexidine.

The position of the needle tip in a particular anatomical structure (transverse abdominal muscle, internal oblique abdominal muscle, external oblique abdominal muscle; within the peritoneal cavity or subcutaneous) will be recorded. After that gel injection will be made. The injection of the gel will be performed by surgeon with experience of performing inguinal hernia repair. However this technique demands approbation on animal (rabbits) and then can be transfered on the humans.

6. Conclusion

Inguinal hernia repair is one of the most common pediatric surgical procedure worldwide. During the last 10 years, laparoscopic surgery has rapidly invaved the pediatric surgical practice. The hopes associated with introduction of a laparoscopy in treatment of pediatric inguinal hernias didn't come true. Unexpectedly, but the randomized, single-blinded, prospective repair between elective laparoscopic and open repair of unilateral inguinal hernia in children showed that recovery and surgical outcome were similar [28]. Besides, laparoscopic repair significantly increased the postoperative time and operative room time.

Injection implants can be regarded as a self-sufficient non-surgical alternative for correction of inguinal hernia in children. No doubt, materials of such kind must be safe and effective, and respond to a number of requirements: biocompatibility, non-toxicity, long-term effect, absence of antigenic properties and pyrogenic reactions. The injection method is excellent alternative to open and laparoscopic methods of treatment of inguinal hernia in children which use an anesthesia and an incision for operation performance. The advantages of this technique are that there is no dissection of the spermatic cord and there is no ligation of the IHS. The near future will show viability of this method.

Author details

Yury Kozlov[1*], Vladimir Novozhilov[2], Vitaly Kovalev[3] and Pavel Krasnov[2]

*Address all correspondence to: yuriherz@hotmail.com

1 Department of Newborn Surgery, Pediatric Hospital Irkutsk, Irkutsk State Medical Academy of Continuing Education, Russia

2 Department of Newborn Surgery, Pediatric Hospital Irkutsk, Irkutsk State Medical Academy of Continuing Education, Russia

3 Department of Newborn Surgery, Pediatric Hospital Irkutsk, Russia

References

[1] Sherer LR, Grosfeld JL. Inguinal hernia and umbilical anomalies. Ped Clin North Am 1993;40:1121–1131.

[2] Skandalakis JE, Colborn GL, Androulakis JA, Skandalakis LJ, Pemberton LB. Embryologic and anatomic basis of in- guinal herniorrhaphy. Surg Clin North Am 1993;73:799–836.

[3] Shcheben'kov M.V. Laparoscopic hernioraphy. Endoscopic surgery (Mosk). 1995; 4: 7-9. [Article in Russian]

[4] Takehara H, Yakabe S, Kameoka K. Laparoscopic percutaneous extraperitoneal closure for inguinal hernia in children: clinical outcome of 972 repairs done in 3 pediatric surgical institutions. J Pediatr Surg. 2006;41:1999-2003.

[5] Ozgediz D, Roayaie K, Lee H, et al., Subcutaneous endoscopically assisted ligation (SEAL) of the internal ring for repair of inguinal hernias in children: report of a new technique and early results. Surg Endosc. 2007;21:1327-1331.

[6] Steigman CK, Sotelo-Avila C, Weber TR. The incidence of spermatic cord structures in inguinal hernia sacs from male children. Am J Surg Pathol 1999;23:880–885.

[7] Chen LE, Zamakhshary M, Foglia RP, et al. Impact of wait time on outcome for inguinal hernia repair in infants. Pediatr Surg Int 2009;25:223–227.

[8] Schier F. Laparoscopic surgery of inguinal hernias in children: initial experience. J Pediatr Surg 2000;35:1331–1335.

[9] Schier F. Laparoscopic inguinal hernia repair: a prospective personal series of 542 children. J Pediatr Surg 2006;41:1081–1084.

[10] Montupet P, Esposito C. Laparoscopic treatment of congenital inguinal hernia in children. J Pediatr Surg. 1999;34:420–423.

[11] Prasad R, Lovvorn HN, Wadie GM, et al. Early experience with needlescopic inguinal herniorrhaphy in children. J Pediatr Surg. 2003;38:1055–1058.

[12] Endo M, Watanabe T, Nakano M, et al. Laparoscopic completely extraperitoneal repair of inguinal hernia in children: a single-institute experience with 1257 repairs compared with cut-down herniorrhaphy. Surg Endosc. 2009;23:1706–1712.

[13] Shalaby R, Shams AM, Mohamed S, et al. Two-trocar needlescopic approach to incarcerated inguinal hernia in children. J Pediatr Surg. 2007;42:1259–1262.

[14] Chan KL, Tam PK. Technical refinements in laparoscopic repair of childhood inguinal hernias. Surg Endosc. 2004;18:957–960.

[15] Miyano G, Yamataka A, Kato Y, et al. Laparoscopic injection of Dermabond tissue adhesive for the repair of inguinal hernia: short- and long-term follow-up. J Pediatr Surg. 2004;39:1867-1870.

[16] Kato Y, Yamataka A, Miyano G. Tissue adhesives for repairing inguinal hernia: a preliminary study. J Laparoendosc Adv Surg Tech A. 2005;15:424-428.

[17] Testini M, Lissidini G, Poli E, et al. A single-surgeon randomized trial comparing sutures, N-butyl-2-cyanoacrylate and human fibrin glue for mesh fixation during primary inguinal hernia repair. Can J Surg;53:155-160.

[18] Bisenkov L.N., Bikhodzhin R.Sh. The endoscopic treatment of bronchial fistulas by submucosal injections. Vestn Khir Im I I Grek. 2005;164:38-41. [Article in Russian]

[19] Bisenkov L.N., Bikhodzhin R.Sh. Prophylaxis and treatment of primary insufficiency of bronchial stump after pneumonectomy. Khirurgiia (Mosk). 2007;1:59-65. [Article in Russian]

[20] Osipov I, Lebedev D, Sosnin E, et al. Our experience in endoscopic treatment of vesico-ureteral reflux in children. Arch Ital Urol Androl. 2005;77:146-148.

[21] Fedorova V.N., Dirsh A.V., Borchunova E.N. Tissue reactivity to the injection of different types of polyacrylamide gels. Regenerative surgery. 2004; № 2. Electronic journal: http://www.reg-surgery.ru/home.html. [Article in Russian].

[22] Luks FI. Gasless laparoscopy in infants. The rabbit model. J Pediatr Surg 1995;30:1206–1208.

[23] Marana R, Luciano AA, Muzii L, et al. Laparoscopy versus laparotomy for ovarian conservative surgery. A randomized trial in the rabbit model. Am J Obstet Gynecol 1994;171:861–864.

[24] Hurd W. A comparison of the relative risk of vessel injury with conical versus pyramidal laparoscopic trocars in a rabbit model. Am J Obstet Gynecol 1995;173:1731–1733.

[25] Ordoñez JL, Domínguez J, Evrard V, et al. The effect of training and duration of surgery on adhesion formation in the rabbit model. Hum Reprod 1997;12:2654–2657.

[26] Molinas CR, Cabral CR, Koninckx PR. Effect of the diameter of the endoscope and of surgeon training on the duration and quality of laparoscopic surgery in a rabbit model. J Am Assoc Gynecol Laparosc 1999;6:447–452.

[27] Willschke H, Marhofer P, Bosenberg A, Johnston S, Wanzel O, Cox SG, Sitzwohl C, Kapral S. Ultrasonography for ilioinguinal/iliohypogastric nerve blocks in children. Br J Anaesth 2005;95:226–30

[28] Denny NM, Harrop-Griffith W. Location, location, location! Ultrasound in regional anaesthesia. Br J Anaesth 2005;95:1–2

[29] Koivusalo AI, Korpela R, Wirtavuori K, et al. A single-blinded, randomized comparison of laparoscopic versus open hernia repair in children.
Pediatrics 2009;123:332–337.

Section 3

Special Types of Groin Hernias

Chapter 6

Strangulated Inguinal Hernia

Evangelos P. Misiakos, George Bagias,
Nickolaos Zavras, Panagiotis Tzanetis,
Paul Patapis and Anastasios Machairas

Additional information is available at the end of the chapter

http://dx.doi.org/10.5772/57379

1. Introduction

An inguinal hernia is an abnormal protrusion of intra-abdominal tissue through a fascial defect in the groin. When a part of bowel which is inside the hernia sac becomes obstructed, there may initially be no interference with blood supply. This case results in a strangulated inguinal hernia, in which gangrene of the contents of the sac has been occurred. Strangulated inguinal hernia is a life-threatening condition which requires urgent surgical intervention. Historically, the prominence of "adhesive bands" as a cause of intestinal obstruction was already known, and was also the main historical cause of small intestinal obstruction before the advent of anesthesia. The descriptive history of hernias can be traced back through the centuries to Hippocrates and the knowledge of the catastrophic effects of incarceration of a hernia dates back to immemorial times. Celsus had referred many interesting historical incidences and he was also the first to describe the surgical techniques for the correction of recurring hernias. Of course, these procedures were very brutal compared to modern techniques, involving various techniques of cautery or caustics [1].

The modern era of thoughtful anatomical and surgical approach to hernia restoration dates back to the beginning of the nineteenth century with Sir Ashley Cooper's and Antonio Scarpa's illustrated monographs in England and in Italy respectively. It is interesting that the life threatening problem of strangulated inguinal hernia was occasionally successfully managed by the simple process of resecting the ischemic part of the bowel, leaving what amounted to a double-barreled enterostomy. Undoubtedly, few patients survived the debilitating effects of small bowel fistula but occasionally intestinal continuity was spontaneously re-established by retraction of the open ends of the bowel and gradual closing of the external fistula. Some of the well-known surgeons of the nineteenth century, such as Gimbernat (1793), Richter (1778),

Camper (1801), Hesselbach (1806) and Scarborough (1809), contributed to the anatomy and clinical findings associated with hernias. There was a limit, however, to what could be accomplished surgically until the introduction of antisepsis, and anesthesia techniques, so subsequent surgeons such as Bassini, Halsted, Billroth, Marcy and others defined the various types of surgical approach to abdominal wall hernias, up to 1880.

2. Anatomy

In the groin, an indirect inguinal hernia is caused when obliteration of the processus vaginalis (the peritoneal extension which accompanies the testicle in its descent into its final position, the scrotum) fails to occur. The hernia sac which has been formed passes through the internal inguinal ring, a defect in the transversalis fascia, between the anterior iliac spine and the pubic tubercle. The sac may extend partway along the inguinal canal, or it can pass through the external inguinal ring, a defect medially in the external oblique muscle, above the pubic tubercle. When the hernia sac reaches fully into the scrotum is called *complete hernia*. The hernia sac and the spermatic cord are invested by the cremaster muscle which is just an extension of internal oblique muscle's fibers [2].

A direct inguinal hernia however, is caused by a weaknes or defect in the floor of Hesselbach triangle. The Hesselbach triangle is defined inferiorly by the inguinal ligament, laterally by the inferior epigastric arteries, and medially by the conjoined tendon. Usually, the transversalis fascia, which forms the floor of Hesselbach triangle, is weakened, though a discrete defect in the fascia may occasionally occur. This type of direct inguinal hernia has distinct borders, thus it is more possible to incarcerate [2].

At this point, we need to mention some anatomic structures, which are important, not only for understanding the pathophysiologgy of hernias, but also for understanding the surgical techniques being used. The conjoined tendon is a fusion of the medial aponeurosis of transversus abdominis and internal oblique muscles, that passes along the inferolateral edge of the rectus abdominis muscle and attaches to the pubic tubercle. The inguinal ligament is formed by the lowermost border of the external oblique aponeurosis, and it passes between the pubic tubercle and the anterior iliac spine. The Cooper ligament is a strong, fibrous band that extends laterally for about 2.5 cm along the iliopectineal line on the superior aspect of the superior pubic ramus. Finally, the iliopubic tract, parallel to inguinal ligament, is a band of connective tissue that starts form the iliopsoas fascia, crosses below the internal inguinal ring, and inserts into the superior pubic ramus, in order to form the Gimbernat ligament.

3. Pathophysiology

The majority of inguinal hernias are indirect hernias. As we mentioned above, an inguinal hernia is formed when the processus vaginalis cannot obliterate, and a direct inguinal hernia is caused when the floor of Hesselbach triangle is weakened. An indirect hernia may dilate the

http://dx.doi.org/10.5772/57379

internal ring and displace or attenuate the inguinal floor. Then the peritoneum may protrude on either side of epigastric vessels, to form a combined direct and indirect hernia, which is called *"pantaloon hernia"*. Contents of this hernia can be part of small intestine, omentum, peritoneum, bladder, and part of colon.

The appearance and progression of a hernia is caused by the increase of intra-abdominal pressure. Many conditions are responsible for this increase. Marked obesity, abdominal strain from heavy exercise, cough, constipation with straining at stool and prostatism with straining on mictutition are some of the common reasons of intra-abdominal pressure's increase. Cirrhosis with ascites, chronic ambulatory peritoneal dialysis and chronically enlarged pelvic orgaans can also contribute. Last but not least, advanced age and chronic debilitating disease can result to transversalis fascia (which forms the floor of Hesselbach triangle) debilitation.

The *strangulation of inguinal hernia* implies interference with the blood supply associated with an obstruction, which may not necessarily be complete. In most cases, it occurs as a complication of intussusception, torsion, volvulus, or any other form of closed-loop obstruction. Interference with the blood supply may occur either from twisting of the bowel on the mesentery or from distension of an obstructed closed loop. It has been pointed out that there is a distinction between long, medium (8±20 inches), and short loop strangulated obstruction. Medium strangulated loops usually result to toxic shock syndrome by the formation of exotoxins of Clostridium welchii, and short loops tend to perforate and cause peritonitis. The contents of the hernia sac can be only ileum, only omentum, ileum with omentum, and rarely only colon, ileum with colon, colon with omentum, testicle, appendix, urinary bladder, Meckel's diverticulum, and preperitoneal tissue.

4. Epidemiology

The incidence rate of strangulated inguinal hernia varies between 0.29 and 2.9 %. The mortality rate also ranges between 2.6 to 9 %, but Tanaka et al[3] have shown that a delay of 12 h increased significantly intestinal resection rate. Needless to say, the delay in diagnosis can also affect the length of hospital stay and hospital costs. Moreover, mortality risk is seven times higher in cases after emergency strangulated inguinal hernia surgery and 20 times higher if bowel resection was undertaken. Strangulated hernias are more frequently seen in elderly patients, and their prevalence in the over-60-year-old population has been reported to be 9.8 % compared with 1.8 % for younger patients; morbidity and mortality rates are 55 and 15 %, respectively, for patients over 65 years in case of herniorrhaphy in emergency. In addition, it has been reported that advanced age in the patients with strangulated inguinal hernia is considered as a prognostic factor of surgical or medical postoperative complications. The relation between mortality and age is understandable, poor risk being related to both intestinal necrosis and systemic complications of more dubious control in emergency circumstances.

5. Diagnosis

5.1. Risk factors

Many habits, conditions and diseases have been accused of development of an inguinal hernia. Patients with abnormal collagen metabolism have an increased risk, due to transversalis fascia debilitation. This fact is substantiated by the higher incidence of inguinal hernias in patients with aortic aneurysm. Abnormality in collagen metabolism can be familial, and studies have revealed families with increased incidence rates of hernias. Smokers have also an abnormal collagen metabolism, as a result smoking is almost certainly considered as a risk factor. Another risk factor is a patent processus vaginalis. Chronic coughing in patients with chronic obstructive pulmonary disease (COPD) seems to be a risk factor, as it contributes to an increase of intraabdominal pressure. Ascites in terms of hepatic cirrhosis and peritoneal dialysis can increase the risk of inguinal hernia or a recurrent hernia. Although physical work is not a risk factor, some studies revealed that long-term and heavy work does increase the risk of hernias [3]. Needless to say that, the patient should be questioned, if it is possible, about these factors. This would help a lot to an early and a safer diagnosis.

Inguinal hernia is a known complication after radical retropubic prostatectomy, whether if it is open or laparoscopic, and has been reported to occur in 7–21% of patients. Other types of lower midline incision surgery as well could promote the development of postoperative inguinal hernia, such as a low (cosmetic) incision for appendectomy, which can disrupt the shutter mechanism and increase the risk of an inguinal hernia. Surgeons should be aware of this important postoperative complication and prophylactic surgical procedures must be evaluated to address the problem.

5.2. Signs and symptoms

As we mentioned above, it has been reported that a delay in diagnosis of 12 h or more, increases significantly morbidity and mortality [4]. This fact points out the importance of the early diagnosis. Strangulated hernia should be regarded as a possible diagnosis in cases of acute small bowel obstruction, especially when no previous laparotomy has been carried out. The first diagnostic tool is the physical examination of the patient. The most common presenting clinical findings for emergency admission are an irreducible mass in the abdominal wall and localized pain (Fig. 1). Patients may have also signs and symptoms of mechanical bowel obstruction, as well as metabolic disorders, such as breath odor, constipation, diarrhea, vomiting and inability for gas exit. Duration of symptoms prior to admission can be from a few hours, up to several days. Significant concomitant medical illnesses can also be found in some cases, though essential hypertension and cardiovascular disorders are considered to be the commonest problems seen. The palpation of the infected area can provide additional information. A punctilious palpation of the inguinal area is needed, in order to locate the hernia site. In the majority of cases, the physical examination establishes the diagnosis of strangulated hernia, and no further examination is needed. The diagnosis of inguinal hernia can be established by physical examination with a sensitivity of 74.5–92% and a specificity of 93%.

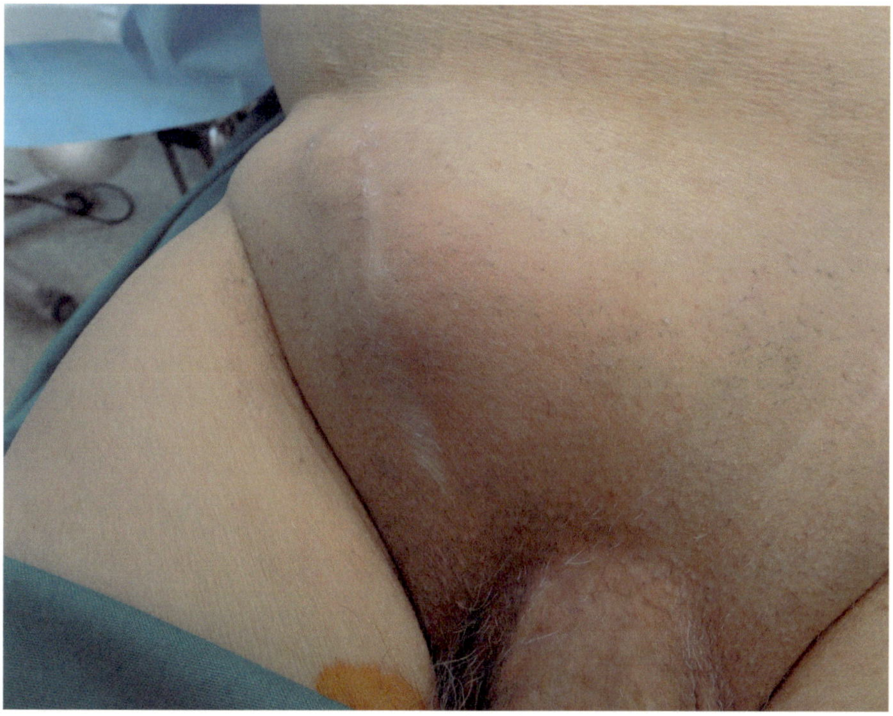

Figure 1. Strangulated recurrent hernia 2 years after a mesh repair. Local swelling, redness, edema and tenderness are the main local signs.

5.3. Imaging examinations

Although they are considered to be rare, there are some cases in which the hernia is occulted, particularly in obese patients, where a small part of the small intestine is strangulated. In these cases, the physical examination cannot establish the diagnosis of strangulated inguinal hernia by itself, and further imaging examinations are carried out. An ultrasonography of the lower abdomen can be performed, after patient's metabolic stabilization, but its sensitivity is low. A computed tomography is another diagnostic tool, with low specificity, but it is useful in the rare case of involvement of the urinary bladder. MRI can also be performed, and is capable for revealing the inflammatory site, and the bowel obstruction, which occurs in strangulated hernias. MRI's sensitivity is 94.5% and specificity is 96.3%. Herniography is also safe, sensitive (100%) and specific (98–100%) imaging examination [4]. Imaging findings are taken into account in combination with physical examination's findings and the general condition of the patient, and the diagnosis is established.

5.4. Laboratory examinations

Although laboratory findings are remarkable, they cannot be used for diagnosis of strangulated inguinal hernia. Hemoconcentration and leucocytosis (especially when is not accounted for by hemoconcentration) can indicate bowel obstruction and strangulation, and so do lactic acidosis, when it does not resolve with volume resuscitation. When the strangulation of small intestine is diagnosed, however, the reason (in this case strangulated inguinal hernia) is not pointed out.

5.5. Surgical diagnostics

A definitive diagnosis of strangulation of the intestine can only be made through surgical exploration. Very little data have been published regarding the laparoscopy and exploratory laparotomy in comparison as a first approach in cases of strangulated groin hernia, when intestinal ischemia is suspected. Although midline laparotomies increase morbidity, due to possible intestinal resection, in some studies, almost the half of overall of midline laparotomies were performed without any intestinal resection [5]. When the patient is older, and there is a big possibility to have a lot of co-morbidities, the laparoscopy or hernioscopy could be of most benefit, avoiding the alternative of a laparotomy. Laparoscopy could help to diagnose bowel ischemia thus decreasing both negative and nontherapeutic laparotomy rates. Once the diagnosis of bowel ischemia is established, laparotomy could be performed. Evisceration, which is a rare occurrence of any incision, is more possible when the patient is old and he/she undergoes an emergency surgery. This complication could be avoided in emergency cases in this advanced aged population by using laparoscopy. Moreover, the decision to perform a bowel resection can be reliably made only by using laparoscopy.

5.6. Differential diagnosis

Strangulated hernia should be distinguished from other conditions which include swelling in the groin. First of all, a differential diagnosis should be made between strangulated inguinal and other types of hernias, such as femoral and incisional hernias. Other cases, in which the patient has groin swelling mass are lymhadenopathy, varicocele, aneurysm, soft-tissue tumor and an abscess, which can be a result of many pathological conditions in the inguinal area. Other relatively rare conditions are endometriosis and several genital anomalies (for example, ectopic testis). Cases that include pain in the inguinal area, but not the typical swelling are adductor tendinitis, pubic osteitis, hip artrosis and bursitis ileopectinea [4].

6. Treatment

A strangulated inguinal hernia, as an incident of acute abdomen, needs emergency surgery. As we mentioned above, the incidence rate of strangulated inguinal hernias is relatively low, because of the high acceptance of the value of elective hernia repair, but it is still a frequent incident of acute abdomen, especially in the elderly patients, in whom the hernia is not always diagnosed until strangulation.

6.1. Anesthesia

The choice between different anesthesia types for inguinal hernia repair is currently under discussion, and it is influenced by patient preferences and his/her medical history. Local anesthesia allows for quick recovery time and, thus, is safe for early discharge in today's increasingly ambulatory surgery era. For patients with increased age or with elevated American Society of Anesthesiologists (ASA) classification (depending on co-existing cardiovascular and/or pulmonary disease), local anesthesia causes much less hemodynamic disorders and it is believed that it is being better tolerated than general anesthesia. Large randomized control studies have shown decrease in overall anesthesia time, urinary retention, and postoperative pain following use of local anesthesia compared to regional and general anesthesia. It has also been indicated that local anesthesia is associated with recurrence rates, but it doubtful whether this increased recurrence rate is a result of local anesthesia, or the use of Lichtenstein repair technique [6].

Needles to say, when herniorrhaphy is performed under local anesthesia, patients still feel the pressure and little pain. These effects can be minimized with the addition of anxiolytic agents. Additionally, the patient must always give consent for the possibility of conversion to general anesthesia, should he or she develop difficulty tolerating the procedure because of anxiety or discomfort.

Commonly used local anesthetics are 0.5-1% lidocaine with epinephrine, or 0.25% bupivacaine, or a combination of these 2 agents in 50:50 mixtures. A field block is applied by injecting along the site of incision, superficial to deep, and lateral to the pubic tubercle, to provide anesthesia to the deeper structures. In order to block the ilioinguinal nerve, an injection is placed just medial to the anterior superior iliac spine. Additional local anesthetic can be injected throughout the procedure. For example, the administration below the fibers of the external oblique aponeurosis, as described by Lichtenstein's group, anesthetizes its 3 major nerves by flooding the enclosed inguinal canal and serves to hydrodissect the underlying ilioinguinal nerve (making it less prone to injury when the aponeurosis is incised). Other techniques, such as epidural anesthesia, have been widely reported, but results depend largely on local expertise.

Elective inguinal hernia repair is considered an aseptic procedure as there is only a <2% surgical site infection rate. Although current data remain controversial, it is suggested (by numerous recent meta-analysis) to use antibiotic prophylaxis when performing a mesh-based repair. Cephalosporins (eg, cefazolin) are commonly administered by the anesthesiologist as a single dose prior to the skin incision. However, a properly funded, prospectively randomized study is still needed to definitively reveal the safest choice of anesthesia.

6.2. Traditional techniques

Traditional surgical repairs, like Bassini and Shouldice techniques are not used very common in elective inguinal hernia repair. However, in an emergency surgery, as in cases of strangulated inguinal hernias, these techniques are preferred from contemporary tension-free techniques, due to high possibility of mesh infection, in tension free techniques. Regardless the choice between traditional and tension-free techniques, the operation begins with an oblique skin incision (or along the Langer lines) approximately 2 centimeter superior to and parallel to the thigh crease, and then the incision is being extended 5 cm toward the anterior superior iliac spine, starting from just lateral to the pubic tubercle. In thin patients, the external ring can actually be palpated just lateral and slightly above the pubic tubercle and should be the medial starting point of incision. Then the dissection is going deeper through the subcutaneous tissue until the aponeurosis of the external oblique is identified. In strangulated hernia the tissues maybe inflamed and edematous, therefore careful dissection of the anatomic structures is mandatory. Along with external oblique aponeurosis, the apex of the inguinal canal and also the external inguinal ring must be identified, before incising the external oblique muscle. The inguinal canal should be entered at its apex. For a correct identification of the apex of the canal, the lower wall of the canal, which is where the external oblique aponeurosis disappears into the fat of the thigh, should be pointed out. Approximately one finger breadth above this point is a good entry site into the canal. The external inguinal ring is also important because the external ring is ultimately the end point of the division to be made in the external oblique aponeurosis and defines the orientation of this cut [6].

Once the external oblique aponeurosis is identified, is thoroughly exposed and a gentle stab incision in its mid-portion along the orientation of its fibers is made. This incision is extended superiorly, and medially downward, through the superficial ring, thus exposing the inguinal canal and the cord structures. Afterwards comes the circumferentially mobilization of the cord structures off the floor of the canal by working on the pubic tubercle as a fulcrum. With blunt dissection of the index finger in a sweeping and medially encircling fashion, the cord is sufficiently freed, so that the cord structures can be surrounded by a Penrose drain for convenient retraction. This allows exposure of the inguinal floor and protects the cord structures. Then, an examination of the anteromedial aspect of the cord should be made, for an indirect component of the hernia. Separating the cremasteric muscle along its fibers often facilitates this. The cremasteric muscle fibers must be dissected carefully with slow electrocautery coagulation, as the cut muscle fibers tend to bleed. If an indirect hernia is present, the sac is dissected off the cord structures, down toward its base at the internal inguinal ring, until it is comfortably invaginated into the preperitoneal space. This is preferably achieved without division of the sac. However, if necessary, as with certain large hernias, the sac can be entered carefully and examined for visceral contents, and then divided with a high ligation. The peritoneal fluid within the sac should be sucked and sent for culture. If there is ischemic bowel inside the sac it should be resected promptly and anastomosed with an end-to-end manner. Occasionally there may be only strangulation of a portion of the greater omentum or strangulation of a portion of the sac itself, which maybe the cause of local discomfort and pain (Fig. 2). Direct hernias, which protrude through the inguinal floor at the Hesselbach triangle, are similarly dissected away from the cord structures toward their base and then are inverted below the transversalis fascia.

Closure of the defect and buttressing of the inguinal canal floor can now be performed. The Bassini technique is widely used, but the Shouldice technique is considered to be better, in terms of recurrence, is not usually used, because of the more extensive dissection, and a belief that the skill of surgeons is important as well. The Bassini repair is a technique in which the surgeon sutures the conjoined tendon to the inguinal ligament, which slides the patient's own muscles together to cover the hole in the abdominal wall and repair the hernia. The spermatic cord remains in its normal anatomic position under the external oblique aponeurosis. The surgeon closes the incision with a stitch known as the simple interrupted suture pattern, a

http://dx.doi.org/10.5772/57379

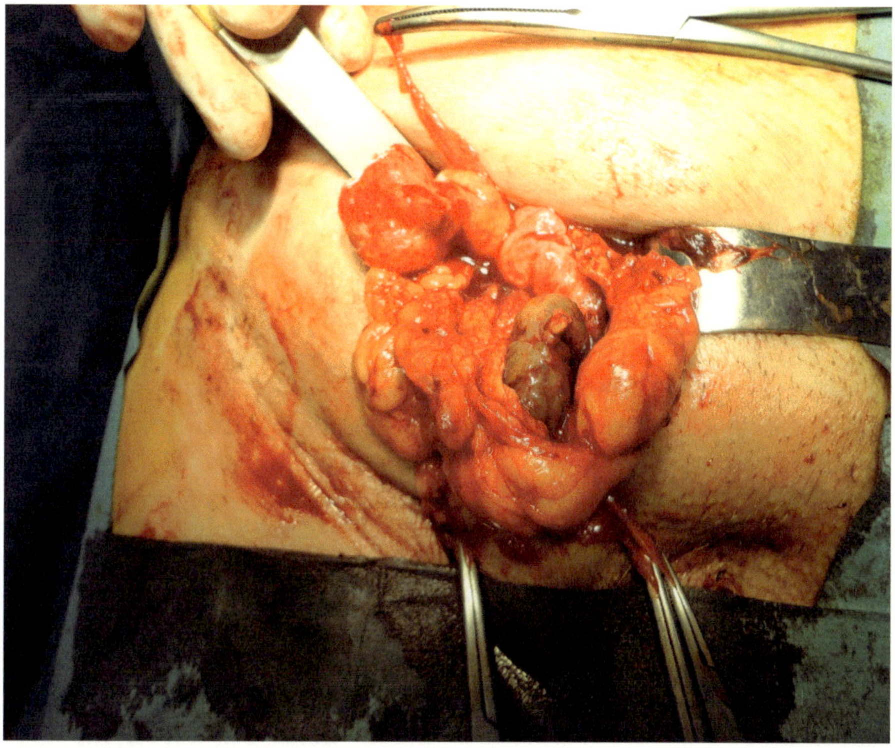

Figure 2. After opening of the subcutaneous tissue, a gangrenous portion of the sac and the adjacent preperitoneal tissue was revealed, which was resected.

speedy stitch that allows for surgery to be complete in approximately one hour. Bassini's original technique yielded outstanding results for a pure tissue technique; however, problems occurred when surgeons failed to open the posterior wall. So, a new operation, known as the "modified" or "North American" Bassini was introduced. By not opening the posterior wall, the wall tissue was damaged in its most medial portion by sutures placed under tension, and recurrences resulted, primarily in the pubic tubercle area. Thus, the failure of this operation in its first year was more likely due to an overlooked second hernia or to poor surgical technique, rather than a metabolic or tissue defect that might predispose to recurrent hernia.

The Shouldice technique (it is also known as ilio-inguinal incision) begins with the ligation of superficial veins. Afterwards, comes the same procedure as described above. The reconstruction in Schouldice technique is achieved by continuous suturing using 2.0 or 3.0 polypropropylene sutures; starting medially, not through the periosteum of the pubic tubercle. Suturation of the inferior edge of the fascia transversalis (Thomson's ligament) to a fold of the anterior side of the conjoined tendon ('white line') is being made, until the internal ring is constricted (in order to allow passage for the spermatic cord and point of tweezers). Then comes the second layer after including cremaster stump with the same thread to the iliopubic tract (inferior edge of the inguinal ligament). The third layer begins laterally, with the closure of the conjoined tendon to inguinal ligament. Original Shouldice has a fourth layer in the same plane. Finally, the reapproximation of the external oblique aponeurosis is achieved with a running 3-0 polyglactin suture; at that stage the surgeon must be careful for the underlying ilioinguinal nerve. Reapproximation of the Scarpa fascia is followed with interrupted 3-0 polyglactin suture and then a running subcuticular closure of the skin with 3-0 poliglecaprone suture. The operative site is cleaned and sterile dressings are applied

6.3. Tension-free techniques

The Lichtenstein repair is widely accepted as the tension-free technique of choice. The operation starts again with medial incision as possible, for good exposure of the tubercle of pubic bone and rectus sheath. The superficial veins are ligated and the external oblique is cleaved, just like the traditional operation (with caution of the ilioinguinal nerve). The spermatic cord is surrounded and the posterior wall is assesed. Cremaster does not need to be excised unless hypertrophic, thus, leaving an unacceptably wide internal ring. The hernia sac is dissected until inside the internal ring, and then it can be reduced (which is the preferable option), transected, or resected. If necessary, the surgeon sutures a large direct hernia tension-free with continuous soluble sutures until a flat posterior wall has been created with a normal internal ring. All nerves should be preserved in principle, but it is advised that if a nerve is damaged or interfers with the palcemnet of mesh it should be resected. Special attention to the iliohypogastric nerve should be paid; this nerve may lie under the mesh, but preferably not against a sharp edge. In that case the prosthesis is cut to the size it needs to be, because it is obvious that dividing a nerve is better than causing neuralgic pain. Polypropylene mesh 7x9x14 cm is applied (trimming is often necessary) with a 2-cm overlap at the pubic tubercle. Then the prosthesis is sutured continuously with polypropylene sutures 3.0 starting 2 cm mediocranially from the pubic tubercule on the lateral rectus edge and then on the inguinal ligament to the internal ring. An incision in the mesh is made on 1/3 of the lower side until just medial to the spermatic cord. And both flaps of the prosthesis are sutured, overlapping on the lateral side to the inguinal ligament with one polypropylene suture; upper flap over the lower flap. The cranial edge of the mesh is also stabilized with one or more sutures (which may be soluble) to the aponeurosis of the internal oblique, avoiding muscle in order to avoid injury to the intramuscular segment of the iliohypogastric nerve. Again particular attention should be paid in order not to entrap nerves by suturing. Mesh must lie tension-free (domed) after removal of the wound spreader. The closure procedure is the same as in the Shouldice technique. In women, it is important to preserve the round ligament and the ilioinguinal nerve (like the spermatic cord). If both structures are cut, it is not necessary to create flaps in the mesh.

6.4. Endoscopic technique

Endoscopic technique has been used rarely in the management of strangulated inguinal hernias, but lately, even more surgeons prefer that technique. In the endoscopic repair (or extraperitoneal approach TEP) the bladder must be empty before the operation. An incision (2 cm) is made just under and next to the umbilicus until inside the anterior rectus sheath. The preperitoneal space is opened with the finger and, if needs be, a balloon (optional) is inserted, up to the pubic bone. The surgeon insufflates with gas, under camera control, and replaces the balloon with blunt balloon or Hasson trocar. The patient is during the procedure in Trendelenburg position. Then, identification of os pubis, Cooper's ligament, epigastric vessels and internal ring takes place. Next, the surgeon dissects with a second trocar (5 or 10 mm in medial line) the lateral space until ASIS and inserts a third trocar (5 mm). The lateral hernia sac is dissected from the spermatic cord which is put aside over 5–7 cm. Polypropylene prosthesis with dimensions 15x9x15 or 10x9x15 cm is inserted and it is draped over the abdominal wall with plenty of overlap for all potential hernia defects. Finally, the surgeon desufflates carefully and removes instruments while holding the peritoneal sac 'inside' the mesh.

6.5. Choice of the most suitable technique

Lately, the use of prosthetic material for inguinal hernia repair has increased dramatically. Tension-free repairs have gained popularity not only for elective or recurrent hernias but also for complicated inguinal hernia repairs as well. Inguinal hernia mesh repair according to Lichtenstein "tension-free" technique has gained great acceptance from the surgeons all over the world, showing efficacy to consolidate the posterior wall of the inguinal canal and to reduce postoperative pain and recurrence risk due to tension on suture lines. Recent clinical trials on tension- free anterior repair of inguinal hernia using a mesh revealed that the immediate postoperative complications were rare and always minor, and rate of long-term recurrence is very low (0.5%) [7].

The presence of a strangulated inguinal hernia cannot be considered a contraindication for the use of a prosthetic mesh, although the use of traditional repairs, such as the Bassini repair in strangulated inguinal hernia is a common practice. Lichtenstein hernioplasty can be successfully used not only as an elective operation but also as an emergency operation for incarcerated inguinal hernia with a good outcome, with a low risk of the local infectious complications and a decently low rate of postoperative complications. However, the outcomes of emergency Lichtenstein hernioplasty were inferior to the outcomes of elective Lichtenstein hernioplasty [8]. Wound infection is a potential complication of all hernia repairs and an infection involving an inserted mesh may result in chronic groin sepsis, which usually necessitates complete removal of mesh. Along with the catastrophic effects of a groin sepsis, removal of mesh would potentially result in a weakness of the repair and as a result, a recurrent hernia. It has been proved however that hernia recurrence following mesh removal for chronic groin sepsis, was not a common phenomenon, and the explanation of that fact is that the strength of a mesh repair lies mostly in the fibrous reaction evoked within the transversalis fascia by the prosthetic material rather than in the physical presence of the mesh itself. Of course, when there is established deep infection, there should be no unnecessary delay in removing an infected mesh in order to allow resolution of chronic groin sepsis. However, that procedure has a relative risk of bowel injury.

Surgical techniques and implanted materials are crucial to the results and costs associated with hernia repair considering that specific mesh materials are related to specific complications. Polypropylene meshes are ideal for use in contaminated or potentially contaminated fields. The macroporous structure of the meshes of polypropylene, with pores of diameter larger than

70 micronmeters, allows contact among the bacteria, which measures almost one micrometer in diameter, and the cells of the immune system, granulocytes and macrophages, with a diameter of 15–20 micronmeters, which is significant for the recovery from infections [7]. The use of antibiotic prophylaxis for tension-free mesh herniorrhaphy may contribute in lowering the incidence of postoperative mesh infection, although there is little direct clinical evidence supporting this fact, and it is not officially recommended.

At this time, a few randomized studies comparing tension-free repairs and classical techniques have been performed, and the available data are considered to be low [9]. It is known that mean operative time and postoperative hospital stay were significantly longer for modified Bassini technique in comparison with tension-free repair, but postoperative complication rate and recurrence rate did not differ significantly between the two operations, according to the latest studies. It is important that in the majority of cases where tension-free repair has been chosen, no mesh had to be removed. Postoperative wound infection rate following Lichtenstein technique is not by far different from that following Bassini technique.

Recurrence rate in cases where a Bassini repair has been performed is approximately 20% and the worst results were observed with direct hernias (29% recurrence) when compared with indirect ones (16% recurrence). Moreover, the use of slowly absorbable suture material in the Bassini technique was reported to result in a high recurrence rate. Also, long-term (12–15 years) recurrence rate following Bassini repair is around 33% [7]. In conclusion, it seems that tension-free repair has lower recurrence rate, and the risk of mesh infection is not as important as it was believed to be during the past decades. Further randomized studies must be carried out, in order to ensure this fact

7. Complications

Postoperative complications are not uncommon after strangulated inguinal hernia repair. Identification of risk factors can be used in order to establish a high-risk group of patients, who are more likely to have a strangulated inguinal hernia. As we mentioned above, advanced age is the most important predisposing factor, as the reserve capacity of the older individual to compensate for stress, metabolic derangement, and drug metabolism is increasingly low. Functional disability occurs faster and it is more difficult to remediate. Some type of complication is encountered in almost half of patients older than 65 years and in 25% of younger patients who have undergone a strangulated inguinal hernia repair. The most frequent serious complications are pulmonary diseases and cardiovascular disorders. Pneumonia is not uncommon, as well as acute exacerbation of chronic obstructive pulmonary disease. Heart failure, coronary artery disease and cardiac arrhythmia are the most frequent complications from the cardiovascular system. Gastrointestinal bleeding, and hepatic failure (in existing cirrhosis) can been found in patients after strangulated hernia repair [10].

Local wound complications are seen in one third of overall patients, Wound infections, hematoma, seroma, and wound dehiscence are some of the most significant wound complications. Urinary retention has been reported in some cases, after the removal of urinary catheter.

Reoperations are not frequent. The causes of reoperations are necrosis of strangulated bowel, evisceration of the bowel, and small bowel obstruction by adhesions. Postoperative mortality has been reduced during the last years, and deaths are usually happening in patients over 65 years who have significant coexisting illness. The causes of death were the following: respiratory failure (which is common between patients with chronic obstructive pulmonary disease), sepsis, which is associated with resection of necrotic bowel in reoperations, and multiorgan failure.

It is doubtful whether there is a significant difference between indirect and direct inguinal hernias in terms of strangulation rate. Postoperative complications have been found by some studies to be more commonly in patients with hernia more than 10 year. Late hospitalization is generally considered to be an important factor for bowel resection and subsequent morbidity and mortality [11]. Usually, the cause of delay in admission is through the patients fault, but a wrong diagnosis can also result in delay of treatment.

Concomitant diseases in patients with incarcerated groin hernias have been reported to be associated with poor outcome, affecting not only the morbidity, but also the mortality rate. The length of hospital stay was also encountered to be longer in patients with concomitant diseases. The ASA class considers the patients' comorbidity and acute physiological disturbance. It has been reported that high ASA score was found to be an independent predictor of gangrenous bowel [12]. A significantly longer hospital stay and a significantly higher morbidity in elderly patients with ASA class III or IV who underwent emergency hernia repair was also reported.

The effect of anesthesia on the outcome of hernia repair has also been examined in the literature [13]. As we mentioned before, it is believed that general and spinal anesthesia were associated with higher rates of postoperative complications, but this fact is not widely accepted.

8. Recurrent inguinal hernia

Recurrent groin hernias are a special complication of strangulated inguinal hernia repair and they are more difficult and hazardous to repair. The frequency of recurrent groin hernias observed after a treatment of strangulated inguinal hernia varied from 10% through 30%. The time to recurrence varies; it is believed to be approximately 25 years, but around 5.6% of recurrences appear during the first postoperative month, and 39.1% of overall recurrent hernias appear during the first year.

The mechanisms of recurrence after a repair are difficult to identify, especially when the recurrence is late, and the previous treatment technique is unknown. Even during the reoperation, the previously used procedure is often not identifiable. Incorrect technique is responsible for most recurrences during the first postoperative year. Examples include not dissecting or not finding a sac, leaving too long a peritoneal "stump", incorrect closure of the hernia orifice, as demonstrated by the frequency of indirect recurrences, and suture under tension, which is most involved in direct recurrences. We previously mentioned that some techniques are more likely than others to lead to a recurrence. These include totally pre- or retrofunicular repairs. Large hernias recur twice as often as small ones, and careless management results in a recurrence. Extended dissection or traumatic sutures may change a contractible inguinal wall into a fibrous wall exposed to progressive rupture. Other risk factors, independent of the quality of the operation, are the patient's general condition and age, abdominal wall weakness, and obesity. The most dangerous factors are postoperative sepsis and chronic cough. It used to blame early activity or return to work for recurrence, but this has been turned down lately, as 80% percent of recurrent hernias are independent of heavy work [14].

Recurrences after prosthetic repair result exclusively from technical mistakes and, thus, appear during the first postoperative year. During the postoperative course, seromas and hematomas must be distinguished from recurrent hernias. The classic clinical signs can be confirmed by ultrasonography. Recurrence rate of strangulated inguinal hernias is high, and it is strongly correlated with the surgical technique. Moreover, technical mistakes during the procedure may worsen this rate. The surgeon must be very careful about the choice of treatment method, considering the predisposing factors that may be present.

Author details

Evangelos P. Misiakos, George Bagias, Nickolaos Zavras, Panagiotis Tzanetis, Paul Patapis and Anastasios Machairas

*Address all correspondence to: misiakos@med.uoa.gr

3rd Department of Surgery, University of Athens School of Medicine, Attikon University Hospital, Athens, Greece

References

[1] McDermott WV Jr. Incarcerated and strangulated hernia. Surg Clin North Am. 1966 46: 789-96.

[2] Skandalakis JE. Embryologic and anatomic basis of inguinal herniorrhaphy. 1993 73:799

[3] Tanaka N, Uchida N, Ogihara H, Sasamoto H, Kato H, Kuwano H. Clinical study of inguinal and femoral incarcerated hernias. Surg Today 2010; 40:1144-7

[4] Simons MP, Aufenacker T, Bay-Nielsen M, Bouillot JL, Campanelli G, Conze J, De Lange D, Fortelny R, Heikkinen T, Kingsnorth A, Kukleta J, Morales-Conde S, Nordin P, Schumpelick V, Smedberg S, Smietanski M, Weber G, Miserez M. European

Hernia Society guidelines on the treatment of inguinal hernia in adult patients. Hernia 2009 13: 343–403.

[5] Romain B, Chemaly R, Meyer N, Brigand C, Steinmetz JP, Rohr S. Prognostic factors of postoperative morbidity and mortality in strangulated groin hernia. Hernia. 2012 16: 405-10.

[6] Stoppa RE. The treatment of complicated groin and incisional hernias. World J Surg. 1989 13: 545-54

[7] Elsebae MM, Nasr M, Said M. Tension-free repair versus Bassini technique for strangulated inguinal hernia: A controlled randomized study. Int J Surg. 2008 6:302-5.

[8] Papaziogas B, Lazaridis Ch, Makris J, Koutelidakis J, Patsas A, Grigoriou M, Chatzimavroudis G, Psaralexis K, Atmatzidis K. Tension-free repair versus modified Bassini technique (Andrews technique) for strangulated inguinal hernia: a comparative study. Hernia. 2005 9: 156-9.

[9] Bessa SS, Katri KM, Abdel Salam WN, Abdel-Baki NA.. Early results from the use of the Lichtenstein repair in the management of strangulated groin hernia. Hernia. 2007 11: 239-42.

[10] Alvarez JA, Baldonedo RF, Bear IG, Solís JA, Alvarez P, Jorge JJ. Incarcerated groin hernias in adults: presentation and outcome. Hernia. 2004 8: 121-6

[11] Brittenden J, Heys SD, Eremin O Femoral hernia: mortality and morbidity following elective and emergency surgery. J R Coll Surg Edinb 1991 36:86–88

[12] Golub R, Cantu R Incarcerated anterior abdominal wallhernias in a community hospital. Hernia 1998 2:157–161

[13] Young DV Comparison of local, spinal, and general anesthesia for inguinal herniorrhaphy. Am J Surg 1987 153:560–563

[14] Deveney KE. Hernias & other lesions of the abdominal wall. Current diagnosis and treatment. 2012 724-36

Chapter 7

Sliding Inguinal Hernias

Andrzej L. Komorowski, David Domínguez Usero,
José Ramón Martín-Hidalgo Rodil and
Jorge Morán-Rodríguez

Additional information is available at the end of the chapter

http://dx.doi.org/10.5772/58223

1. Introduction

A sliding inguinal hernia is a protrusion of a retroperitoneal organ through an abdominal wall defect. Frequency of sliding hernias is estimated at 3-8% of all elective operations of inguinal hernias. Sliding hernias are supposed to be more anatomically challenging for a surgeon than an uncomplicated non-sliding inguinal hernias. The anatomical and physiological concept of sliding inguinal hernia is frequently misunderstood by surgeons of all levels of experience. Not infrequently, any inguinal hernia that is big enough or has any organ (e.g. small intestine) inside its sac is referred to as sliding hernia. In this chapter we will try to clarify the pathology behind the sliding inguinal hernia and explain its correct management.

2. History and current classification

Sliding hernias are known to surgeons for almost three centuries. Since the first description by Italian surgeon and anatomist from Pavia, Antonio Scarpa in 1809 [1] they were feared as a complicated surgical conditions. The main obstacle in surgical approach to this type of hernias was-and still is-the fact that part of the hernia sac is in reality a retroperitoneal organ thus, during opening of the sac an inadverent damage to a vital organ can be made. The advance of anatomical knowledge and evolution of surgical technique allowed for a better understanding of this entity. With the better understanding of pathological anatomy of the sliding hernia various classification systems have been introduced. Currently the best and most frequently used classification of sliding hernias is the one by Robert Bendavid [2]. Bendavid divides the sliding inguinal hernia into three anatomical variants depending on the size of the sac and its relation to the retrperitoneal „slided" organ. Type I is defined as any hernia in which part of the peritoneal sac is made up by the wall of a viscus (Figure 1). Type II is defined as any hernia containing a retroperitoneal viscus and its mesentery, in which the mesentery forms part of the wall of the peritoneal sac (Figure 2). In type III the sliding hernia consists on a protrusion of a viscus itself, and the peritoneal sac is very small or even absent. This last variant is an extremely rare finding and accounts for approximately only 0.01% of all inguinal hernias. Figure 1 and Figure 2 depict in a schematic way two most common types of sliding inguinal hernias according to Bendavid. We strongly advocate the use of this classification in everyday practice as it enables surgeons to better understand the concept and hence better plan the operation of a sliding inguinal hernia.

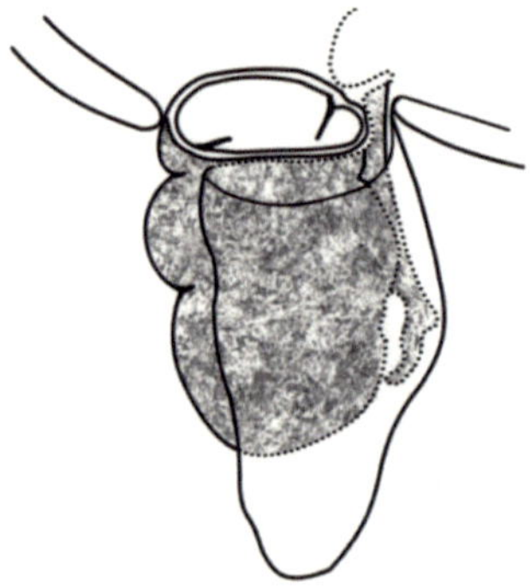

Figure 1. Schematic drawing of Bendavid Type I sliding inguinal hernia. The posterolateral aspect of the hernia sac is made up of the caecum and ascending colon. This type of sliding inguinal hernia accounts for almost 95% of all sliding inguinal hernia cases. The most common contents are: sigmoid, caecum, appendix (by dr Jerzy W. Mituś based on Bendavid [2]).

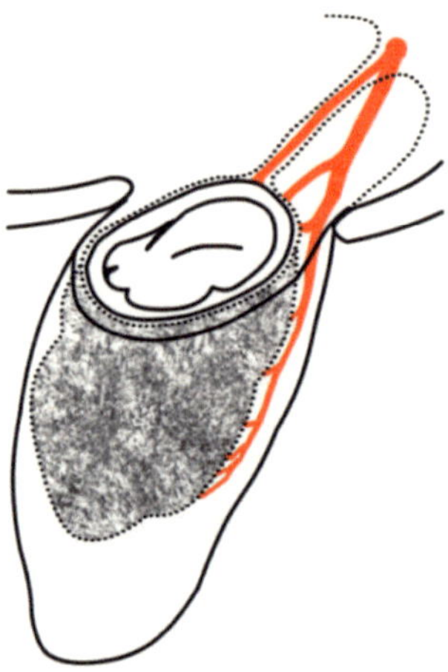

Figure 2. Schematic drawing of Bendavid Type II sliding inguinal hernia. In this hernia the mesentery forms part of the posterior wall of the sac and part of the anterior wall of the caecum forms part of the posterior wall of the sac. This type of sliding inguinal hernia accounts for about 5% of all sliding inguinal hernia cases. The most common contents is sigmoid (by dr Jerzy W. Mituś based on Bendavid [2]).

http://dx.doi.org/10.5772/58223

3. Clinical presentation

Sliding hernia is quite a common finding in infant girls: up to 20% of all hernias in this group of patients are sliding hernias containing ovary and fallopian tube [3]. In the adult population almost all cases of sliding hernias are seen in men [4, 5] with only isolated reports of sliding inguinal hernias in women [6]. Frequency of the sliding hernia in adults was historically estimated at around 6–8% of all hernia cases [4] but more recent report by our group estimate its frequency at 3.4% [5]. Most probably it is due to the fact that today's hernia patient present with smaller hernias with shorter duration of symptoms or even before the onset of symptoms. The sliding hernias tend to occur in older patients that develop symptoms for quite a long time. In one of the biggest series of inguinal sliding hernias, published by Ryan in 1956, the average age of patients with sliding hernia was 60 years[4]. On the other hand, in our recently published series the average age of patients presenting with sliding inguinal hernia was estimated at 70 [5] and is higher that some current series reporting a mean age of 63 years [7]. The mean duration of symptoms in the series by Ryan was 12 years, 6 years in our series and in some reports it can be as low as 9 months [8]. As one can see the age of patients and duration of symptoms have dropped over the time, but still are higher than the same numbers describing current general population of inguinal hernia patients. The mean age of an inguinal hernia patient is estimated at 53 years and the mean duration of symptoms at 2.8 years for UK patients [9]. These numbers can be quite different in some selected groups of patients as in the aforementionned report by Adams which cited only 9 months median duration of symptoms of a sliding inguinal hernia patients in his Australian patient population [8].

It is very rare to establish preoperative diagnosis of a sliding inguinal hernia as there are no particular clinical signs indicating the possibility of sliding hernia. Older patients with big hernias, presenting with a long history of inguinal lump are the group most likely to have a retroperitoneal organ protruding into the hernia sac [5]. In the literature there are rare case reports of preoperative diagnosis of a sliding inguinal hernia containing urinary bladder based on a plain abdominal x-ray showing urinary bladder calculi within the groin [10]. However, in the vast majority of cases the diagnosis is made after the hernia sac is opened (as seen on Figure 3). If a surgeon does not open a hernia sac, a small sliding hernia can be easily overlooked. If the sac is manipulated gently this should not have any influence on the outcome of surgery in therms of early and late complications. As in the current practice it is becoming increasingly rare for surgeons to routinely open an inguinal hernia sac, a number of sliding hernias can undergo surgery without being recognized as such.

Interestingly, important percentage of sliding inguinal hernias can present as complicated cases with almost 12% of all sliding hernias presenting with intestinal obstruction to the emergency department [7]. This finding is obviously absent in reports on sliding hernias that are dealing only with elective inguinal hernia cases [5].

Another possible form of acute presentation of a sliding inguinal hernia is a perforation of the cancer of the sigmoid colon forming part of the hernia sac. This complication, although extremely rare implies a change in opertive strategy as correction of the hernial defect falls behind the priorities of resolving perforation and performing adequate oncologic colon resection [11].

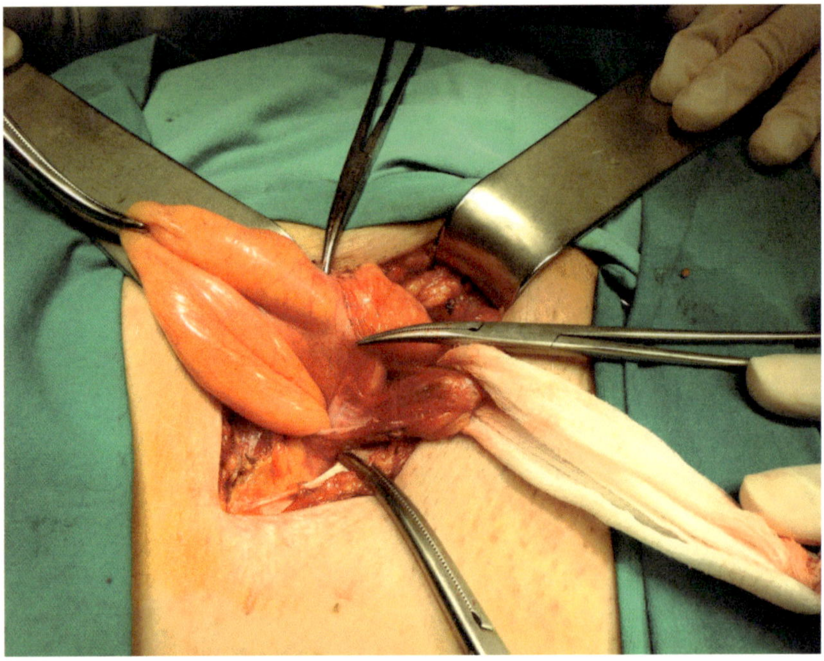

Figure 3. Opening of an inguinal sliding hernia sac. (Servicio de Cirugia General, Hospital Virgen del Camino, Sanlucar de Barrameda-Cadiz, Spain)

4. Management

Traditionally sliding hernias were considered difficult to operate on. For an inexperienced or non-prepared surgon even today it can pose quite a challenge [8]. One of the main reason why sliding inguinal hernia used to be considered such a difficult operation, was that in previous decades it was customary to aim at the excision of a whole peritoneal hernia sac and high ligation of a remaining stump. Given that in a sliding hernia a part of the sac is formed by the retroperitoneal organ the risk of injury of that organ was indeed higher. Currently the excision of a sac is not considered mandatory. Gentle dissection of the sac allows to perform tension free repair as in any inguinal hernia operation [2].

In the recently published paper our group have tried to identify all sliding inguinal hernias in a series of almost 500 elective hernia operations [5]. During the study period we have recorded 16 cases of a sliding inguinal hernias (incidence 3.4%). All patients with sliding hernias were male. The dominant hernia side was left (69%) similarly to the majority of the published series e.g. in the series by Patle [7] it reached 76%, with sigmoid colon being the most common slided organ. Other slided organs were retroperitonel appendix, caecum and urinary bladder and all were Bendavid type I hernias (Figure 1).

The opening of the sac and control of its content was performed in all our cases to confirm the diagnosis of a sliding hernia. However, some authors suggest that in case of a doubt as to the nature of the sac it is advisable not to open it, as the sac itself may prove to be intestinal or urinary bladder wall [2]. As mentioned before it is not necessary to open all hernia sacs. In our series the opening of all suspected sacs was indeed performed but only due to the experimental nature of the study. All patients in our experience were operated using prosthetic mesh with or without plug. This approach can be seen as a bit risky but once again we should stress that gentle dissection and clear anatomy are the keys to the success of the operation and the safe use of the same prosthetic materials that we routinely use for our inguinal hernia patients. We have indeed not seen any intestinal complications in our group of sliding inguinal elective hernias. The only postoperative complications that might be attributable to the use of mesh in this series are wound infection and seroma formations. However, none of these complications required explanations of the mesh [5]. In the long term follow-up we have not observed any rise in the abdominal symptoms that could be attributable to the use of prosthetic material close to the serous surface of the retroperitoneal organ that formed the hernia sac.

The laparoscopic repair of a sliding inguinal hernia is possible, however it requires important technical skills. Even in the hands of the most experienced laparoscopic hernia surgeons the conversion to open procedure can be necessary in as much as 10% of all cases [7].

5. Conclusion

The fundaments of sliding inguinal repair are meticulous, gentle dissection and identification of all anatomical structures. Opening of the sac is not necessary. A surgeon operating according to these principles and supported by a wide range of prosthetic material is in a far better situation than his surgical predecessors. The good operating technique and the use of modern prosthetic materials should allow us to have the same risk of early and late complications after operating on a sliding and non-sliding inguinal hernia.

Acknowledgements

The authors wish to thank dr Jerzy W.Mituś from Kraków, Poland for the preparation of the Figures 1 and 2.

Author details

Andrzej L. Komorowski[1], David Domínguez Usero[2], José Ramón Martín-Hidalgo Rodil[2] and Jorge Morán-Rodríguez[3]

1 Department of Surgical Oncology, Maria Skłodowska-Curie Memorial Cancer Centre, Kraków, Poland

2 Department of General Surgery, Hospital Virgen del Camino, Sanlucar de Barrameda, Cadiz, Spain

3 Department of General Surgery, Hospital San Juan Grande, Jerez de la Frontera, Cadiz, Spain

References

[1] Scarpa A. Sull'ernie: memorie anatomo-chirurgiche. Milan: Stamperia Reale, 1809-1820

[2] Bendavid R. Sliding hernias. Hernia 2002; 6:137-140.

[3] Kaneko K, Ando H, Tsuda M. New surgical procedure for sliding inguinal hernia repair in female infants and girls. J Am Coll Surg 2002; 194: 544-546.

[4] Ryan EA. An analysis of 313 consecutive cases of indirect sliding inguinal hernias. Surg Gyn Obst 1956; 102:45-58.

[5] Komorowski AL, Moran Rodriguez J, Kazi R, Wysocki WM. Sliding Inguinal Hernias. Int J Surg 2012;10(4):206-208

[6] Ozkan OV, Semerci E, Aslan E, Ozkan S, Dolapcioglu K, Besirov E. A right sliding indirect inguinal hernia containing paraovarian cyst, fallopian. Arch Gynecol Obstet 2009;279:897e9.

[7] Patle NM, Tantia O, Prasad P, Khanna S, Sen B. Sliding inguinal hernias: scope of laparoscopic repair. J Laparoendosc Adv Surg Tech A. 2011 Apr;21(3):227-31.

[8] 8. Adams RA, Wysocki AP. Outcome of sliding inguinal hernia repair. Hernia. 2010 Feb;14(1):47-9.

[9] Browne J, Jamieson L, Lewsey J, van der Meulen J, Copley L, Black N. Case-mix & patients' reports of outcome in Independent Sector Treatment Centres: Comparison with NHS providers. BMC Health Serv Res 2008; 8:78.

http://dx.doi.org/10.5772/58223

[10] Chi Fai Ng A, Leung AKC, Robson WLM. Urinary bladder calculi in a sliding vesical-inguinal-scrotal hernia diagnosed preoperatively by plain abdominal radiography. Adv Ther 2007; 24:1016-1019.

[11] Tan A, Taylor G, Ahmed T. Perforated sigmoid colon carcinoma in an irreduciblein-guinoscrotal hernia. Ann R Coll Surg Engl. 2013 Oct;95(7):125-6

Chapter 8

Groin Pain in Athletes — Sports Hernia and Osteitis Pubis

Baki Ekçi and Tahsin Beyzadeoglu

Additional information is available at the end of the chapter

http://dx.doi.org/10.5772/58621

1. Introduction

Sport is all forms of usually competitive physical activity. This intense activity might result with injuries associated with the overload to the muscles and joints. During competitive sports activities made under tough conditions, the load over the groin is often excessive. It was suggested that groin injuries are more common in sports that require repetitive fast twisting and turning movements (eg, soccer and hockey). It is caused by muscular imbalances and weaknesses that result in an uneven distribution of forces. In this chapter, common reasons for the groin pain in athletes, namely sports hernia and osteitis pubis will be extensively reviewed and discussed.

It is estimated that groin pain occurs in 5% to 28% of athletes [1]. On the other hand, activity restricting lower abdomen and groin pain is frequent in some sports, such as soccer, accounting for 10% to 13% of all injuries per year [2]. The prevalence of groin pain may be higher in some types of sports activities involving repeated kicking and rapid change of direction, such as soccer, tennis, football, and ice and field hockey. In these higher competitive sports, the incidence may rise to 5–7% of all injuries [3]. The patients presenting with groin pain are usually highly competitive athletes pushing the limits, runners and players who are willing to achieve college auditions or top league. This is a common problem that can be career-limiting or career ending for a player and remains a serious clinical challenge for the sports physician and treating surgeon.

The most common causes of groin pain in athletes are injuries to the adductor longus, iliopsoas, and rectus femoris muscles and injury to the inguinal floor. These conditions may cause hyperextension injury, insertion tendinitis and direct hernia or bulge. Other causes of groin pain include ilioinguinal neuralgia, osteitis pubis, genitourinary sources (prostatitis, epididymitis, urethritis, and hydrocele), nerve compression, bursitis, and arthritis of the hip.

Sports hernia is the overflow of the internal organs and intestine through a particular weak point. This condition is not a complete herniation. However, due to the overuse of the muscles, this pushing movement might cause recurring pain at that area. Since, this condition occurs at every repeating movement, the athlete will eventually avoid making such movements thereby exerting negative influence on his performance. So-called Gilmore's groin, athletic pubalgia, sports hernia, incipient hernia, and posterior abdominal wall deficiency, the term "sports hernia" (athletic pubalgia), is described as a condition of chronic exercise-related supra-inguinal groin pain, which is associated with an incipient direct bulge of the inguinal wall whenever the abdominal muscles contract forcefully. Sports hernia is also termed as external oblique tear-occult hernia, nonspecific attenuation of the inguinal floor with cord lipoma, internal ring weakness, occult hernia, not true hernia-injury at the rectus insertion, muscular injury due to overexertion of the inguinal region, medial inguinal floor injury, deficiency of the posterior inguinal wall [4-11]. This condition has been poorly understood by the clinicians [12-15].

First described by Beer in 1924, osteitis pubis is a noninfectious, self-limited inflammatory condition of the symphysis pubis involving the adjoining pubic bones, the perichondrium, and the periosteum [16-19]. Osteitis pubis is known as one of the causes of groin pain, which is associated with the overuse related to kicking and running resulting in shearing stress at the symphysis. Thus, it is very common among athletes. It is also typical in sports comprising a lot of sprinting and sudden changes of direction, such as running, basketball, soccer, ice hockey, and tennis [20, 21]. On the other hand, it has been reported to complicate a variety of pelvic surgeries, including abdominoperineal resection, inguinal herniorrhaphy, endoscopic resection of the prostate, after anterior colporrhaphy, retropubic urethropexy, even after periurethral collagen injection and endoscopic inguinal hernia repair resulting from attachment of the stapler to os pubis [22, 23].

The clinician must also consider that athletes with groin pain may have other orthopaedic and nonorthopaedic potential causes of the groin pain. The differential diagnosis is various. Muscle strain (adductor, rectus, iliopsoas), osteitis pubis, stress fracture, avulsion fracture, hip joint injury, nerve entrapment, and lumbar radiculopathy can be orthopaedic problems, such as classic hernia, appendicitis, diverticulitis, irritable bowel syndrome, adhesions, urinary tract infection, prostatitis, testicular pain, varicoceles, endometriosis, ovarian cyst, and round ligament entrapment can be non-orthopaedic conditions [24, 25].

2. Mechanism of injury

The aetiology of both conditions has not been completely understood. However, excessive physical activity is assumed as the etiological factor since these conditions are quite common among athletes. Athletes with a previous groin injury history, elder athletes, players having inactive periods out of the season, and the players making sports involving only a particular part of their muscles have a higher risk [26, 27]. Various factors have been suggested for the mechanism of sports hernia. Athletic pubalgia is described as an occult hernia process or an

http://dx.doi.org/10.5772/58621

incipient hernia, with the major abnormality being a defect in the transversalis fascia, which forms the posterior wall of the inguinal canal, and not a muscle tear [2] (Figure 1).

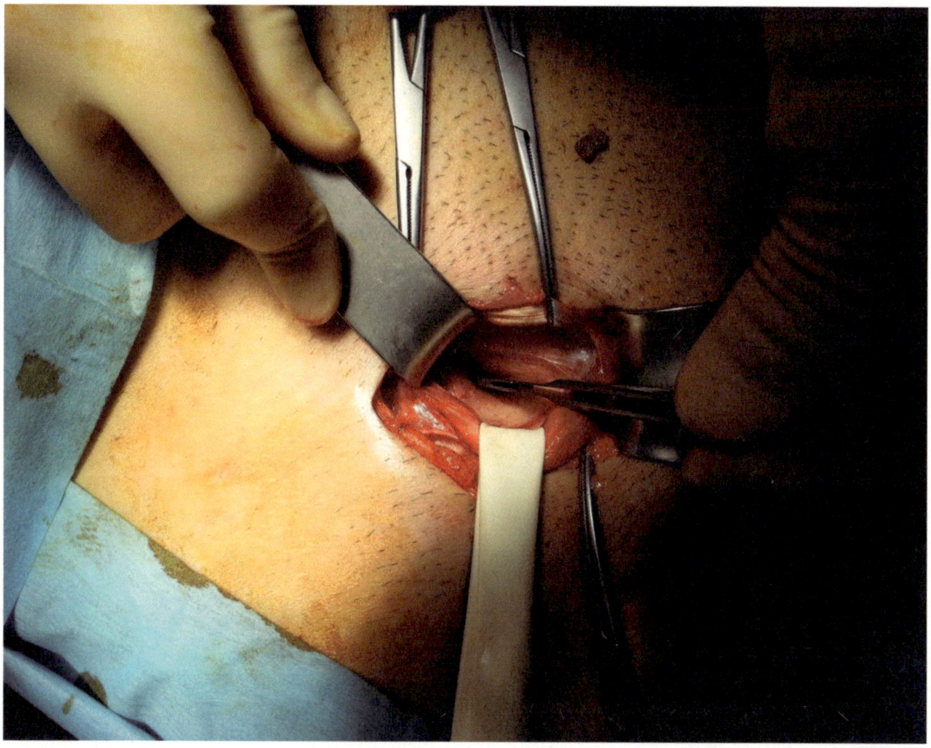

Figure 1. Abnormality being a defect in the transversalis fascia

Gilmore proposed a mechanism of injury in athletic pubalgia, that was a tear in external oblique aponeurosis, conjoined tendon tears from pubic tubercle and conjoined tendon splits from inguinal ligament (7, 28, 29). Furthermore, Meyers et al. [30] suggested that the primary mechanism for most of these injuries involves hyperextension of the abdomen and/or hyper-abduction of the thigh, and the pain occurs primarily with exertion, often in multiple locations, rarely involving the internal ring. The cutaneous nerves include the iliohypogastric nerve (sensory to the lower abdomen), the ilioinguinal nerve (sensory to the groin), and the genital branch of the genitofemoral nerve (sensory to the scrotum and labia)[24]. Muschawek reported that posterior inguinal swelling exerts pressure on genital nerve and this might cause pain [7, 31]. This nerve irritation produces a dull or burning pain that radiates into the inner thigh or scrotum. In addition, external oblique defects traumatize ilioinguinal and iliohypogastric nerves resulting with inguinal pain [30, 32] (Figure 2). As it is understood, this condition cannot be explained with only one mechanism. Muscular imbalances in high performance athletes, coordination disorders, excess weight and continuous training, irregular training are among important factors resulting with groin pain.

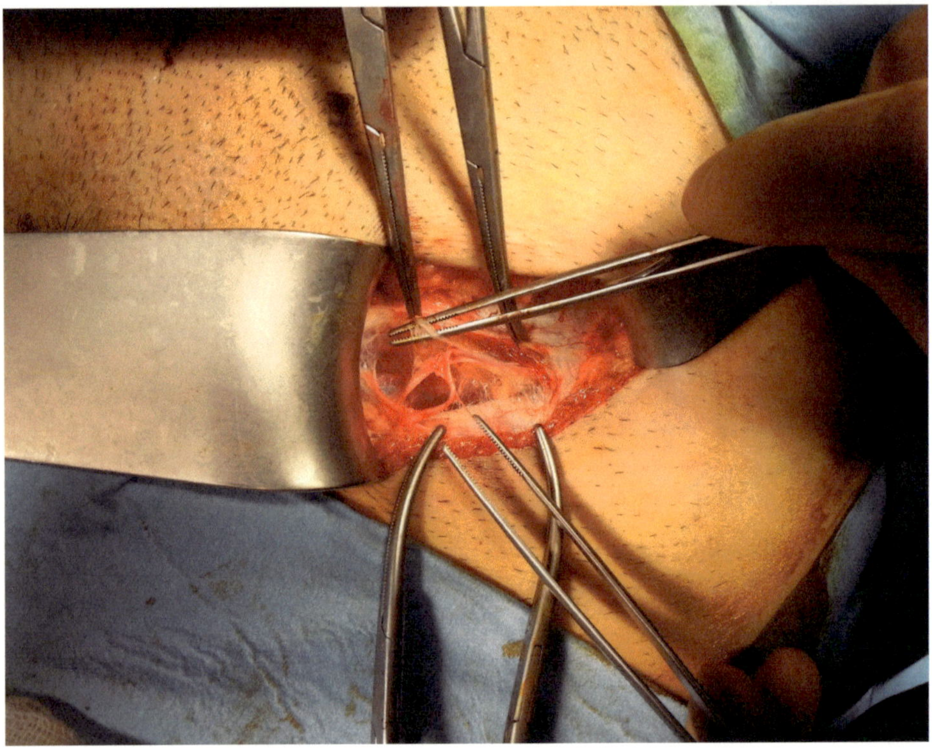

Figure 2. External oblique defects traumatize ilioinguinal and iliohypogastric nerves resulting with inguinal pain

The symphysis pubis is a nonsynovial-lined, amphiarthrodial joint located between the two pubic bones. Biomechanical analysis of the pelvis has revealed that the innominate bones function as arches, thus transferring the weight of the upright trunk from the sacrum to the hips. The exact cause of this condition is unclear; however, it appears that the overuse related to kicking and running results in shearing stress at the symphysis. Traction, micro trauma and instability of the sacroiliac joint and symphysis pubis can be the possible causes of osteitis [19, 33]. The four main hypotheses for the cause of postoperative osteitis pubis include trauma, impaired vascular circulation, trophic bone changes related to a causalgia-like mechanism and infection [17, 20, 34]. Osteitis pubis is the result of intraoperative trauma to the symphysis and its muscular attachments either from surgical instruments or retractors [16, 22, 34]. In Marshall-Marchetti-Krantz procedure, in which sutures are placed directly into the periosteum or cartilage of the symphysis pubis, osteitis pubis is uncommon [35, 36].

3. Physical examination

In sports hernia, moderate pain and discomfort in the region of inguinal area associated with exertion, sneezing and coughing are mostly noted. These are usually abated with rest. The presenting symptom develops during exercise, aggravated by sudden movements. Pain persists after a game, abates during a period of lay-off, but returns on the resumption of sport [37]. In physical examination, physician should evaluate inguinal hernia, pubis, rectus abdominis, hips and adductor muscles. In addition, local tenderness at the conjoined tendon, pubic tubercle, or inguinal canal might be observed. On examination, the athlete usually has pain with passive stretch of the adductors and pain on adduction against resistance. The athlete will often have pain with resisted sit-ups and resisted hip adduction [37]. Coughing, sneezing, and other Valsalva-type maneuvers often worsen the pain. Over the conjoined tendon or medial inguinal canal, the distal rectus insertion, pubic tubercle, and/or adductor origin points are tenderness [38]. The most common finding is a dilated, tender internal inguinal ring, true inguinal hernia is rarely found (1, 6, 10). But, the physician should exclude the presence of an inguinal or femoral hernia. The onset of complaints, the types of movements causing pain, measures for avoiding pain, time of resting and acts for coping with pain should be learned in details. A true herniation is rarely seen in this group of patients; the base of inguinal canal is weakly detected and might be sensitive [39, 40].

The diagnosis of osteitis pubis is based on typical clinical symptoms and abnormal radiographic findings. Common clinical symptoms are suprapubic pain, difficulty, and pain with ambulation. Pain can occur while walking, radiating to the perineal, suprapubic region [41, 42]. The anterior portion of the pelvis and the adductor muscles are tender and spasm may accompany. Pain is usually radiates to the suprapubic area and the adductor surfaces of the thighs and it usually begins ten days to two months after an operation upon the urinary bladder [43]. Pain is the primary symptom associated typically with difficulty in ambulation and the characteristic "waddling gait" [42, 44]. Symptoms may develop from 1 to 8 weeks after the initiating event. The duration of the signs and symptoms is related to the severity of the inflammation and the response to therapy after the appropriate diagnosis is established [42]. Laboratory findings may be mild leucocytosis, raised levels of acute phase proteins (fibrinogen, C reactive protein), and increased erythrocyte sedimentation rate.

4. Diagnostic test

Diagnostic tests are required to rule out other pathologies associated with lower abdominal, hip or groin pain. After a complete history and physical exam, the patient should have a complete blood count, urinalysis, and ultrasound of the groin firstly. Diagnostic imaging includes an erect pelvic radiograph (X-ray) with flamingo stress views of the symphysis pubis, real-time ultrasound and, occasionally, computed tomography (CT) scanning and magnetic resonance imaging (MRI), but seldom contrast herniography [25, 37]. The patient is examined with USG while lying in a supine position. A high-resolution linear array transducer of 10 MHz or greater frequency is recommended [15]. Other imaging tests occasionally performed can include nuclear bone scan, limb leg measurement.

A standard athletic pubalgia protocol includes coronal and axial large field-of-view fluid-sensitive, fat-suppressed images that should adequately cover this region and identify the injury and this MRI protocol is generally adequate [45]. Stress fractures, tendon avulsion and hip arthrosis might be detected by x-ray, and ultrasound might show incipient inguinal hernia. If physician suspect bone tumours, hip ring pathologies, spine or retroperitoneal problems may want to see CT. Hip problems and bursitis, MRI be the best choice in determination of aetiology of inguinal pain in sports but it may be normal in sport's hernia [45]. Pelvic MRI might give more detailed information regarding the condition of pelvis and soft tissue, alterations due to edema and stress, muscle tears, adductor muscle groups, and the location of pubis muscle insertions. An advantage of USG assessment is that this method may show the dynamic movements of inguinal floor with the help of Valsalva maneuver. If the results of these tests are negative and the symptoms continue with sports hernia symptoms, a laparoscopic preperitoneal exploration might be carried out [11].

Early in the course of osteitis pubis, radiographs are typically normal [19]. After approximately 6 months, x-rays of the symphysis may show a frayed appearance of the pubic periosteum, loss of cortex, widening, erosions, and sclerosis along the articular border [15, 35]. These findings included erosion, rarefaction, resorption, and sclerosis of the pubic bones. In its early stages, osteomyelitis presents similarly to osteitis pubis and its make the diagnosis difficulty. Close monitoring of patients diagnosed with osteitis pubis is recommended in these patients. If a question about the diagnosis exists, computed tomography-guided pubic bone aspiration for culture is advocated [22]. The athletes who have this disease with normal AP radiographs had bone scans that demonstrated increased radiotracer (99mTc) uptake throughout the area of the symphysis pubis as a characteristic of osteitis pubis. A bone scan, which is more sensitive than radiography, usually shows the increased uptake in the pubic bones on both sides of the symphysis and pubic ramus, often before any radiographic changes are seen [46, 47] [48]. MRI and computed tomography scans can show inflammatory changes in the bone. MRI illustrates joint-space alteration, articular surface irregularity, para-articular marrow edema and extrusions of the symphyseal disk and includes low intensity signal on T1 weighted and a high intensity signal on T2 weighted images [49]. Sclerosis has low intensity signal on both T1 and T2 weighted images [50]. (Figure 3) High-resolution MRI and ultrasound may identify subtle tears and defects within one or more of the structures that inserts around the groin region [15]. MRI appearances in osteomyelitis and osteitis are similar in the initial stages. Both osteitis pubis, an inflammatory disease, and osteomyelitis, an infectious disease, can appear in one patient at the same time. In these cases, biopsy and culture may be necessary to make a differential diagnosis [18, 49].

MRI and ultrasound (US) can be used to exclude co-existing abnormalities in the patients undergoing a groin repair. Bilateral abdominal abnormalities on ultrasound may appear to be a valid marker for inguinal pain and the anatomic injury [51]. According to the location and morphology of the patient medium to high-frequency linear probes can use and colour Doppler examination may be useful. Investigation carried out in dynamic conditions (coughing and the Valsalva maneuver) may important. Additionally US can show the reinforcement positioned in the area of wall weakness after surgery [52]. Posterior inguinal wall deficiency can be demonstrated sonographically, as the contraction of the anterior abdominal wall results in loss of the normal valve-like effect of the canal [15] (Figure 4).

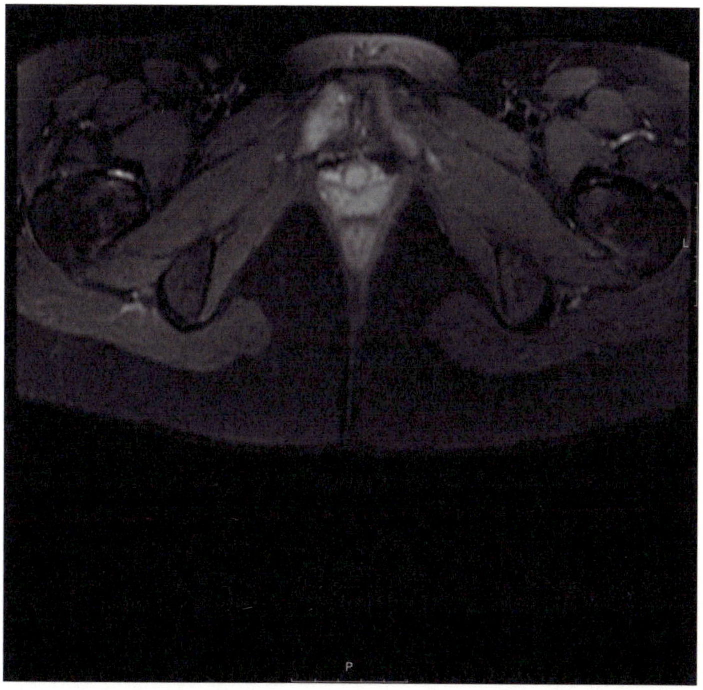

Figure 3. MRI illustrates joint-space alteration, articular surface irregularity, para-articular marrow edema and extrusions of the symphyseal disk and includes low intensity signal on T1 weighted and a high intensity signal on T2 weighted images. Osteitis pubis on the right pubic bone.

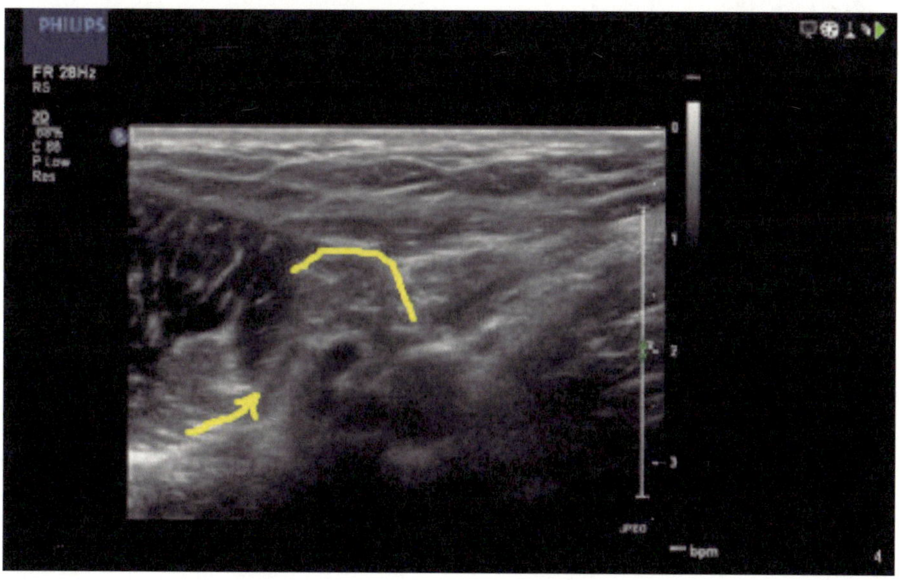

Figure 4. Posterior inguinal wall deficiency can be demonstrated sonographically

5. Management

In both conditions, the first treatment choice is resting and standard conservative treatment. In sports hernia, it is important to determine the movements causing symptoms and avoiding them. Conservative treatments are effective in relieving pain and returning the athlete to normal sports activities. This approach might involve the application of heat or ice, stretching and strengthening exercises, analgesic medications and other physical-therapy interventions. In elective cases, the use of corticosteroids and local analgesics might relieve symptoms. If the symptoms are relieved and under control, slight lower body exercises might be started. This period may last for 6-8 weeks, or occasionally 10 weeks. There is still no consensus on the surgical treatment techniques. Open primary repair, open mesh repair, laparoscopic mesh repair, neurectomy, and adductor tendon relaxation are among the surgical techniques [24]. Mesh repair technique is so-called Lichtenstein hernia repair. In open repair, Muschawek technique, also called minimal repair might be used [24, 31]. A number of different modified repairs of the posterior wall deficiency have also been described [30, 37]. Groin reconstruction operation consists of a Maloney darn hernia repair technique, repair of the conjoint tendon, transverse adductor tenotomy and obturator nerve release [37]. Laparoscopic mesh repair technique is also used. In this technique, synthetic and biological meshes, which have been advocated to reinforce the posterior wall of the inguinal canal, are preferred [53, 54]. Rehabilitation treatment is important in the post-operative course. On the other hand, sutureless tension-free hernia repair with fibrin glue may be the choose for treatment of hernia[55] Rehabilitation programs in which activities are gradually increased in the 5-8 weeks period are utilized. Specific rehabilitation targeted at abdominal strengthening, adductor muscle flexibility, and a graduated return to activity. Rehabilitation may takes about 3 months after surgery [24, 37, 56].

Management of osteitis pubis can be difficult; whether to make conservative treatment or surgical intervention is controversial. Conservative treatment usually involves rest, oral medication with non-steroidal anti-inflammatory drugs, daily use of therapeutic modalities a progressive rehabilitation programme [57-59]. Earlier return to full activity has been reported injection of corticosteroid and local anaesthetic [21, 60]. Complete recovery can take over a few months. Curettage, arthrodesis, wedge resection and wide resection are described for surgical intervention of osteitis pubis [41, 61].

In conclusion, sports hernia and osteitis pubis are particularly common among athletes making sports with excessive load on their muscles that may compromise their professional careers. Being cautious while training and making exercises might be helpful at preventing such injuries. The diagnosis of these conditions might be easily mixed up with the other causes of groin pain. Treatment is substantially conservative or surgical intervention might be preferred in some cases if required.

Author details

Baki Ekçi[1] and Tahsin Beyzadeoglu[2]

1 Yeditepe University, Medical School, Department of General Surgery, Istanbul, Turkey

2 Private Practice of Orthopedics and Traumatology, Beyzadeoglu Sports Medicine Clinic, Istanbul, Turkey

References

[1] Nam A, Brody F. Management and therapy for sports hernia. Journal of the American College of Surgeons. 2008;206(1):154-64.

[2] Litwin DE, Sneider EB, McEnaney PM, Busconi BD. Athletic pubalgia (sports hernia). Clinics in sports medicine. 2011;30(2):417-34.

[3] Kavanagh EC, Koulouris G, Ford S, McMahon P, Johnson C, Eustace SJ. MR imaging of groin pain in the athlete. Seminars in musculoskeletal radiology. 2006;10(3): 197-207.

[4] Fon LJ, Spence RA. Sportsman's hernia. The British journal of surgery. 2000;87(5): 545-52.

[5] Ahumada LA, Ashruf S, Espinosa-de-los-Monteros A, Long JN, de la Torre JI, Garth WP, et al. Athletic pubalgia: definition and surgical treatment. Annals of plastic surgery. 2005;55(4):393-6.

[6] Farber AJ, Wilckens JH. Sports hernia: diagnosis and therapeutic approach. The Journal of the American Academy of Orthopaedic Surgeons. 2007;15(8):507-14.

[7] Muschaweck U, Berger LM. Sportsmen's Groin-Diagnostic Approach and Treatment With the Minimal Repair Technique: A Single-Center Uncontrolled Clinical Review. Sports health. 2010;2(3):216-21.

[8] Paajanen H, Ristolainen L, Turunen H, Kujala UM. Prevalence and etiological factors of sport-related groin injuries in top-level soccer compared to non-contact sports. Archives of orthopaedic and trauma surgery. 2011;131(2):261-6.

[9] Paajanen H. ["Sports hernia" and osteitis pubis in an athlete]. Duodecim; laaketieteellinen aikakauskirja. 2009;125(3):261-6.

[10] Diesen DL, Pappas TN. Sports hernias. Advances in surgery. 2007;41:177-87.

[11] Edelman DS, Selesnick H. "Sports" hernia: treatment with biologic mesh (Surgisis): a preliminary study. Surgical endoscopy. 2006;20(6):971-3.

[12] Akita K, Niga S, Yamato Y, Muneta T, Sato T. Anatomic basis of chronic groin pain with special reference to sports hernia. Surgical and radiologic anatomy : SRA. 1999;21(1):1-5.

[13] Brown A, Abrahams S, Remedios D, Chadwick SJ. Sports hernia: a clinical update. The British journal of general practice : the journal of the Royal College of General Practitioners. 2013;63(608):e235-7.

[14] Shortt CP, Zoga AC, Kavanagh EC, Meyers WC. Anatomy, pathology, and MRI findings in the sports hernia. Seminars in musculoskeletal radiology. 2008;12(1):54-61.

[15] Davies AG, Clarke AW, Gilmore J, Wotherspoon M, Connell DA. Review: imaging of groin pain in the athlete. Skeletal radiology. 2010;39(7):629-44.

[16] Beer E. Periostitis of the symphysis and descending rami of the pubis following suprapubic operations. Int J Med Surg. 1924;37:224-5.

[17] Cibert J. Post-operative osteitis pubis: causes and treatment. British journal of urology. 1952;24(3):213-5.

[18] Gibbon WW, Hession PR. Diseases of the pubis and pubic symphysis: MR imaging appearances. AJR American journal of roentgenology. 1997;169(3):849-53.

[19] Middleton RG, Carlile RG. The spectrum of osteitis pubis. Comprehensive therapy. 1993;19(3):99-102.

[20] Fricker PA, Taunton JE, Ammann W. Osteitis pubis in athletes. Infection, inflammation or injury? Sports medicine. 1991;12(4):266-79.

[21] Holt MA, Keene JS, Graf BK, Helwig DC. Treatment of osteitis pubis in athletes. Results of corticosteroid injections. The American journal of sports medicine. 1995;23(5): 601-6.

[22] Frederick RW, Carey JM, Leach GE. Osseous complications after transvaginal bone anchor fixation in female pelvic reconstructive surgery: report from single largest prospective series and literature review. Urology. 2004;64(4):669-74.

[23] Karray S, Karray M, Zlitn M, Bahri H, Litaiem T, Douik M, et al. [Pubic osteitis after treatment for inguinal hernia. Apropos of 2 cases]. Annales de chirurgie. 1995;49(1): 78.

[24] Minnich JM, Hanks JB, Muschaweck U, Brunt LM, Diduch DR. Sports hernia: diagnosis and treatment highlighting a minimal repair surgical technique. The American journal of sports medicine. 2011;39(6):1341-9.

[25] Swan KG, Jr., Wolcott M. The athletic hernia: a systematic review. Clinical orthopaedics and related research. 2007;455:78-87.

[26] Emery CA, Meeuwisse WH. Risk factors for groin injuries in hockey. Medicine and science in sports and exercise. 2001;33(9):1423-33.

[27] Tyler TF, Nicholas SJ, Campbell RJ, McHugh MP. The association of hip strength and flexibility with the incidence of adductor muscle strains in professional ice hockey players. The American journal of sports medicine. 2001;29(2):124-8.

[28] Gilmore J. Groin pain in the soccer athlete: fact, fiction, and treatment. Clinics in sports medicine. 1998;17(4):787-93, vii.

[29] Sheen AJ, Stephenson BM, Lloyd DM, Robinson P, Fevre D, Paajanen H, et al. 'Treatment of the Sportsman's groin': British Hernia Society's 2014 position statement based on the Manchester Consensus Conference. British journal of sports medicine. 2013.

[30] Meyers WC, Foley DP, Garrett WE, Lohnes JH, Mandlebaum BR. Management of severe lower abdominal or inguinal pain in high-performance athletes. PAIN (Performing Athletes with Abdominal or Inguinal Neuromuscular Pain Study Group). Am J Sports Med. 2000;28(1):2-8.

[31] Muschaweck U, Berger L. Minimal Repair technique of sportsmen's groin: an innovative open-suture repair to treat chronic inguinal pain. Hernia : the journal of hernias and abdominal wall surgery. 2010;14(1):27-33.

[32] Irshad K, Feldman LS, Lavoie C, Lacroix VJ, Mulder DS, Brown RA. Operative management of "hockey groin syndrome": 12 years of experience in National Hockey League players. Surgery. 2001;130(4):759-64; discussion 64-6.

[33] Harris NH, Murray RO. Lesions of the symphysis in athletes. British medical journal. 1974;4(5938):211-4.

[34] Lavalle LL, Hamm F. Osteitis pubis: its etiology and pathology. The Journal of urology. 1951;66(3):418-32.

[35] Kammerer-Doak DN, Cornella JL, Magrina JF, Stanhope CR, Smilack J. Osteitis pubis after Marshall-Marchetti-Krantz urethropexy: a pubic osteomyelitis. American journal of obstetrics and gynecology. 1998;179(3 Pt 1):586-90.

[36] Garcia-Porrua C, Picallo JA, Gonzalez-Gay MA. Osteitis pubis after Marshall-Marchetti-Krantz urethropexy. Joint, bone, spine : revue du rhumatisme. 2003;70(1):61-3.

[37] Garvey JF, Read JW, Turner A. Sportsman hernia: what can we do? Hernia : the journal of hernias and abdominal wall surgery. 2010;14(1):17-25.

[38] Caudill P, Nyland J, Smith C, Yerasimides J, Lach J. Sports hernias: a systematic literature review. British journal of sports medicine. 2008;42(12):954-64.

[39] Cavalli M, Bombini G, Campanelli G. Pubic Inguinal Pain Syndrome: the So-called Sports Hernia. Surgical technology international. 2014;XXIV.

[40] Campanelli G. Pubic inguinal pain syndrome: the so-called sports hernia. Hernia : the journal of hernias and abdominal wall surgery. 2010;14(1):1-4.

[41] Mehin R, Meek R, O'Brien P, Blachut P. Surgery for osteitis pubis. Canadian journal of surgery Journal canadien de chirurgie. 2006;49(3):170-6.

[42] Lentz SS. Osteitis pubis: a review. Obstetrical & gynecological survey. 1995;50(4): 310-5.

[43] Friedenberg ZB. Osteitis pubis with involvement of the hip joint. The Journal of bone and joint surgery American volume. 1950;32(A:4):924-7.

[44] Matsuda DK. Endoscopic pubic symphysectomy for reclacitrant osteitis pubis associated with bilateral femoroacetabular impingement. Orthopedics. 2010;33(3).

[45] Zoga AC, Meyers WC. Magnetic resonance imaging for pain after surgical treatment for athletic pubalgia and the "sports hernia". Seminars in musculoskeletal radiology. 2011;15(4):372-82.

[46] Briggs RC, Kolbjornsen PH, Southall RC. Osteitis pubis, Tc-99m MDP, and professional hockey players. Clinical nuclear medicine. 1992;17(11):861-3.

[47] Burke G, Joe C, Levine M, Sabio H. Tc-99m bone scan in unilateral osteitis pubis. Clinical nuclear medicine. 1994;19(6):535.

[48] O'Kane JW. Anterior hip pain. American family physician. 1999;60(6):1687-96.

[49] Pauli S, Willemsen P, Declerck K, Chappel R, Vanderveken M. Osteomyelitis pubis versus osteitis pubis: a case presentation and review of the literature. British journal of sports medicine. 2002;36(1):71-3.

[50] Andrews SK, Carek PJ. Osteitis pubis: a diagnosis for the family physician. The Journal of the American Board of Family Practice / American Board of Family Practice. 1998;11(4):291-5.

[51] Jansen JA, Mens JM, Backx FJ, Stam HJ. Diagnostics in athletes with long-standing groin pain. Scandinavian journal of medicine & science in sports. 2008;18(6):679-90.

[52] Balconi G. US in pubalgia. Journal of ultrasound. 2011;14(3):157-66.

[53] Ingoldby CJ. Laparoscopic and conventional repair of groin disruption in sportsmen. The British journal of surgery. 1997;84(2):213-5.

[54] Genitsaris M, Goulimaris I, Sikas N. Laparoscopic repair of groin pain in athletes. The American journal of sports medicine. 2004;32(5):1238-42.

[55] Canonico S, Benevento R, Della Corte A, Fattopace A, Canonico R. Sutureless tension-free hernia repair with human fibrin glue (tissucol) in soccer players with chronic inguinal pain: initial experience. International journal of sports medicine. 2007;28(10):873-6.

[56] Biedert RM, Warnke K, Meyer S. Symphysis syndrome in athletes: surgical treatment for chronic lower abdominal, groin, and adductor pain in athletes. Clinical journal of

sport medicine : official journal of the Canadian Academy of Sport Medicine. 2003;13(5):278-84.

[57] Sudarshan A. Physical therapy management of osteitis pubis in a 10-year-old cricket fast bowler. Physiotherapy theory and practice. 2013;29(6):476-86.

[58] Jarosz BS. Individualized multi-modal management of osteitis pubis in an Australian Rules footballer. Journal of chiropractic medicine. 2011;10(2):105-10.

[59] Holmich P, Uhrskou P, Ulnits L, Kanstrup IL, Nielsen MB, Bjerg AM, et al. Effectiveness of active physical training as treatment for long-standing adductor-related groin pain in athletes: randomised trial. Lancet. 1999;353(9151):439-43.

[60] Batt ME, McShane JM, Dillingham MF. Osteitis pubis in collegiate football players. Medicine and science in sports and exercise. 1995;27(5):629-33.

[61] Radic R, Annear P. Use of pubic symphysis curettage for treatment-resistant osteitis pubis in athletes. The American journal of sports medicine. 2008;36(1):122-8.